Shruti

Ayurveda for Well-Being

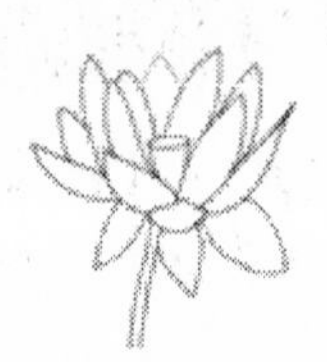

Ayurveda encompasses self-cure or 'Svabhavoparamavada'. It believes that the human body inherently knows its own unique power of self-defence and spontaneous healing against disease. The role of Ayurveda or any medicine is to assist in natural healing faculties.

Shruti

Ayurveda for Well-Being

Aasiya Rizvi

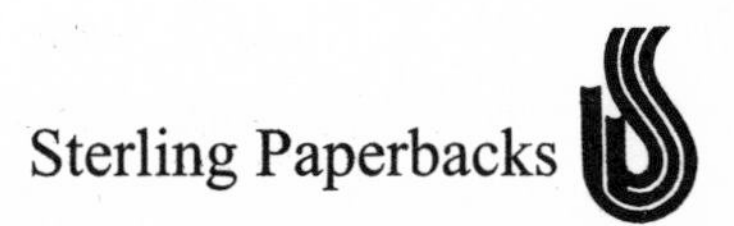

STERLING PAPERBACKS
An imprint of
Sterling Publishers (P) Ltd.
A-59, Okhla Industrial Area, Phase-II,
New Delhi-110020.
Tel: 26387070, 26386209; Fax: 91-11-26383788
E-mail: mail@sterlingpublishers.com
www.sterlingpublishers.com

Shruti: Ayurveda for Well-Being

ISBN 978 81 207 5889 6

Yoga Illustrations:
Artist Kukku Hussain

Printed in India

Printed and Published by Sterling Publishers Pvt. Ltd.,
New Delhi-110 020.

Foreword

Namaste!

My name is Dr Sibi George and I am a traditional Ayurvedic healer. I come from the South Indian State of Kerala. I have over 25 years of experience in the Ancient Indian Ayurvedic Science and Therapies and Massages after having learned from the traditional professional knowledge from my father (Ayurvedic Doctor). I started my career in 1986 as a teacher and a Therapy Practitioner. Now I bring this knowledge to everyone with my treatments.

Aasiya Rizvi and I met several years ago when she was inquiring about some courses and treatments with me. At the time she was also interested in Tibetan Medicine and visiting the Tibetan doctors and the Men Tse Khang Institute for Tibetan Medicine. She was very interested as her family was also connected to Ayurveda. We met in Bhagsunag,Himachal Pradesh, where I am mainly in my clinic during the summer time. During the winter months I am in Kerala as I offer treatments and courses in the clinics.

Ayurveda is one of the great gifts of the sages of ancient India to mankind. It is one of the oldest scientific medical systems in the world with a long record of clinical experience to validate it. However, it is not only a system of medicine in the conventional sense of curing disease. It is also a way of life that teaches us how to maintain and protect health. It shows us how to both cure disease and promote longetivity. Ayurveda treats man as a 'whole' – though at the same time viewing him a combination of body, mind, and soul therefore it is a truly holistic and integral medical system. I am very happy that Aasiya has written this book to share the Ayurvedic way of life with others. She has made a sincere and genuine effort to share her points of view and give light to Ayurveda. This can be very beneficial for everyone in a profound way.

I believe that everyone is looking for peace and health but it will not come to you, you have to bring it to yourself. This is why Ayurveda teaches you that 'Self-Realization' or determining your 'individuality' and constitution in humours is important. It is so essential to recognize yourself. Your bad and good, your positive and your negative egos etcetera. Then accordingly, you can design your life by diet and lifestyle. I really hope that this handbook "Shruti" helps you and guides you to the good bridge.

The word Ayu means all aspects of life from birth to death. The word Veda means knowledge of learning. Thus Ayurveda denotes the science by which life, in its totality, is understood. It is a science of life that delineates the diet, medicines, and behavior that are beneficial or harmful for life. Aasiya has included the main chapters in her book that inform us of what is healthy for us according to Ayurveda. Her book may be used as a handbook of recommendations that can be useful to anyone who is interested in Ayurveda. By reading this book you can get a wonderful idea of what Ayurveda is and also get the important guidelines in a compact form. These guidelines are for preventive medicine and lifestyle and also for general Ayurvedic medicine and treatments.

Ayurveda teaches you more than 68 varieties of Ayurvedic treatment procedures or therapies and has a vast number of Ayurvedic medicinal cures. Some of these main treatments are Pancha Karma, (A comprehensive system of knowledge and practice to purify the body from toxins and restore it to balance with natural law). Usually, a 28-day or more programme is recommended for this .Other therapies are Kizhy, Pizhichill, Dhara, Marma Therapy, Stone Therapy, Ennathoni, and many different types of massages and even more. It can take more than one lifetime to fully embrace all of Ayurveda because there is so much knowledge in it. Experience has always shown that whenever people have come from within India and the West to get treatments from me or to learn about Ayurveda they have always felt the benefits in their lives. Aasiya's book *Shruti* will also bring people to a deeper understanding of Ayurveda and to experience it as wisdom that is not far away but very close to our hearts. I am sure that the reader will enjoy this book and also learn many good things.

'Loka Samastha Suhino Bhvanthu'

'May all be blessed with eternal peace'

Dr Sibi George
Kerala Traditional School of Ayurveda
near Bhagsunag Temple, Bhagsu, HP, India
E-mail: sibi80@hotmail.com, sibi80@gmail.com

Preface

Ayurveda has progressively gained in worldwide recognition as a holistic healing system of medicine and preventive medicine. It is approached as both an alternative and as a complementary medicine. It is often compared with Traditional Chinese Medicine or Tibetan Medicine. It offers a broad array of knowledge in the field of natural healing faculties.

My first meeting with Ayurveda was through my cultural and ancestral heritage. While many of my family members are doctors specialised in their particular fields of medicine, I regularly heard references made to my grandfather who was an Ayurvedic cum Unani doctor. He had studied in Tibbia Medical College in Delhi during the pre-partition time of India and Pakistan after which he founded a centre, the "Dawa Khana" in the province of Sind, Pakistan. He was much admired for his knowledge and healing abilities and authored many books that were dedicated to universities in the area.

Ayurveda is still actively used amongst most families even though many might not be entirely aware of this. The negative aspects of modern life have also affected families in Asia and altered people's lifestyle and manner of relating with life in its totality. In today's Ayurveda we can find a variety of Spas and Massage centres spread across the world. In India there are restaurants that present themselves to serve Ayurvedic meals but are instead serving popular Indian dishes, Ayurveda beauty products, herbal teas and many more products are more readily available to everyone. Several professional Ayurveda clinics and centres have also opened up, there are government hospitals in India, and as time is elapsing, we may find professional doctors and practitioners all over the world.

I began to embrace Ayurveda several years back as I progressively began to meet with the phenomena of holistic medicine. I grew up in pace with modern life, dutifully completing high school, followed by university studies unto office work. I enjoyed the corporate life for a while but recognised that something fundamental was lacking. It was as if the unnatural felt natural. The way of life seemed out of balance with little time left to feed the body in a healthy manner. I instinctively knew there was a gentler way to nourish oneself at a deeper level as well. The only way out of this tempo seemed to be the way inward. I began to contemplate unto a more spiritual path; one that is harmonious with the tunes of nature. This deep inner journey brought me very close to Ayurveda.

I spent many years embracing the sweetness of Ayurveda, researching it and I travelled through India and Pakistan to bring me to a closer understanding of it. I realised that the subject was vast, almost infinite yet very down-to-earth and its true essence lay in its divinity. Ayurveda inspires us to recognise the healthy state of being within ourselves and offers guidelines toward sustenance of good health. It recognises and respects that each living creature is unique and precious.

In feeling that each grain we devour is sacred, each fire we ignite is inextinguishable in essence, and that each shift in a mood we experience is no coincidence but can be a communion with the One, I only ascertained to move even closer to Ayurveda. It is common human folly to forget simple gentle gifts and truths that life is continuously revealing to us. In silence almost everything can be revealed to us. Our cosmic memories can be nurtured and awakened. Through Ayurveda one comes to experience the delicate interconnectedness of life, one realises compassion, love and can reach balance in life.

I received my diploma as an Ayurvedic practitioner from the Eisra College of Ayurveda in the Netherlands. I have lived in the Netherlands since my early teens. This college is affiliated with the Gujarat University in India. The founder of my college, my teacher, Dr Mehta, is a well-renowned doctor and a very loving man who I first met in 1998 prior to my journeys. He founded the first Ayurvedic centre and college in the Benelux and eventually extended his clinics back to India. He has also authored several books, taught hundreds of students and healed many people with diseases like cancer. During my internship in India I met with many, local and international patients. I witnessed a change in pulse – during the daily pulse diagnosis check of patients – and a 'glow of life' gradually re-immersing in patients who were battling with leukaemia and tumours. Each morning, the gardener would collect those parts of plants that were needed to make medicines. The yoga therapist would open-heartedly support in healing people morning and evening and daily Ayurvedic treatments were given in the therapy rooms. Some patients turned to Vedic astrologers and the cook would wipe the sweat of his brow as he persevered to produce Ayurvedic meals each day in accordance to people's constitutions and diseases.

This book *Shruti* gives an overview of what Ayurveda is and offers people a handbook of guidelines and recommendations for better health care and understanding with Ayurveda. It is written in a way for both professionals in the field of Ayurveda as well as for the layman who knows little or nothing about Ayurveda. In addition to this, Shruti also places Ayurveda at the heart of Divine Wisdom. It reflects on how such wisdom is essentially universal and in a way does not belong to any one tradition or culture. Divine wisdom exists in us all and always has across the globe. Perhaps the best gift of Ayurveda to humankind is the recognition and respect that we can all be self-healers. In sharing this book, I hope readers will become even more gentle and loving to themselves and towards their environment. Ayurveda is a gentle and loving way of healing and preventive medicine.

-Author

Acknowledgements

I offer my deep gratitude to Swami Prem Nirmal, Abila Rizvi, Dr Mehta, my parents, Sibi George, Surinder Ghai and Abbas Jaffri for their loving help and much support for the publication of this book. Thank you as well to Kukku Hussain for her art work.

Contents

Table of Figures

Introduction

This book addresses Ayurveda, the wisdom of life received by the rishis or seers of the Indian subcontinent 5000 years ago up to modern times. As much as Ayurveda is an ancient wisdom, it is also timeless knowledge. While some areas in the ancient scriptures are not that relevant in our modern times such as using the hair from the tail of an animal for surgical purposes, other knowledge is of great benefit to us, sacred and indispensible such as daily, seasonal and ethical guidelines for a joyous, healthy and fulfilling life with ourselves and one another.

This book further re-examines the guidelines of Ayurveda for daily, seasonal and ethical routines not just for the region of the Indian subcontinent but also for the western world. In a way Ayurveda came down to Earth from Heaven – metaphorically speaking - to all peoples all over the planet and is the knowledge and science to meet with Heaven and Earth within ourselves. So, one might say there is Ayurveda of Africa, Americas, Europe and we need to remember Ayurveda as the wisdom of life wherever and how so ever we happen to be. Let us remember that wisdom has also been received by the Mayas, Aztecs, Toltecs and the Shamans around the planet and that we are at a very privileged time on Earth where we can manifest together now. When we put all this knowledge together we will notice certain things: The most important thing is that there is something universally common in all these different traditions. This is what we need to connect to in this period of time. We will also notice that there are differences due to local climatic and botanical differences in the foods, animals and plants species around – which is natural.

As a student and practitioner of Ayurveda, I have on one hand felt intrigued and privileged to meet with such sacred knowledge as is Ayurveda yet limited at how this wisdom cannot be easily applied at a holistic level in this modern era. I am in search of how best this wonderful wisdom can be applicable to assist the well-being of mankind. The questions that will be looked at in this book are:

1) Can the daily and seasonal routines described in the Charaka Samhita (i.e. one of the three oldest Ayurvedic scriptures written by Charaka on internal medicine) be applied anywhere in the world?
2) Can the ethical routines described in the Charaka Samhita be applied in our lives today?

At first glance, the answer can be a simple "yes" or "no" yet it is worthwhile to make Ayurveda more pragmatic. This book serves as a guidebook to the wisdom of life for the layman who knows little or nothing about Ayurveda as well as for professionals in Ayurveda who are interested in how it can be adapted in our lives in the present century at a local and global level.

We need to update the principles of Ayurveda in terms of the new environment on the planet which is dominated by the technosphere. A rishi is someone who observes, who is clairvoyant. Today's "rishis" are people who are in sincere good research about what is healthy for us and what is not. The difficulty in this period of time is an overload of information, some of it is contradictory. How does one navigate with this overload of information? For this we can thank the rishis of today for their investigations.

Chapter one introduces Ayurveda as a loving science of how to take care of ourselves. Chapter two briefly introduces yoga and its benefits. Chapter three is about Ayurveda today. Chapters four and five are about daily and seasonal routines followed by Chapter six about diet. Finally, Chapter seven denotes the ethical routine and is followed by the conclusion. There are also appendices at the end of the book with some recipes and properties of gems, metals and colours.

Ayurveda originated in the Himalayan region of the Indian subcontinent but it also includes essential points that are common to all spiritual traditions:

There has been conscious realization that life is a gift which needs our deepest respect and attention for all to go well. We are each the caretaker of our body. It is a temporary event and our bodies are like temples of 'God'.

There has also been an understanding of what it is to be a human. This is deep sacred knowledge of man as a micro and macrocosm.

There has also been an active worship of the sun, moon, earth, stars, wind, fire, water and plants.

An understanding of the music of the spheres and respecting the harmonic order of sound has been a common tradition. The chanting of mantras and sacred sounds and music have always been practices and a direct way to be in harmony with our health and well-being.

Another common spiritual tradition has been the teaching of cosmology (non manifest to manifest, sun, moon, angels, God; Kabbala – Tree of Life, Celtic, Inca, Maya and Aztec). Study of the four directions or 8 directions up down, left right, diagonal, bowing – prostration is common to all wisdom traditions – which is sacred geometry.

There has been the tradition of breath work (controlled breathing with the intent of purification) forceful exhalation, inhalation and taking in of "food that is clean". It is a common alchemical process. Exhaling what is alchemized.

It has been a tradition to connect all the subtle bodies and our physical bodies unto the study of death and knowledge of ourselves as channels. We are receptors of multi-dimensional forms, vibrations, colours, sounds, thought forms and feelings.

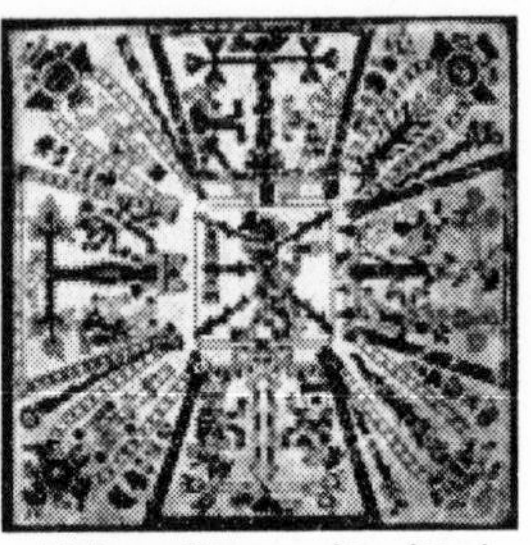

j jFigurejjMayanjSunjGod

The teaching in plant and food knowledge; study of aloe vera (in warm, dry parts of Earth), mint, nettle (Milarepa, for instance almost entirely could only live on nettle), sage, usage of plant perfume, i.e. olfactory science, aromatherapy. Other common nectars from Earth are honey, milk, rain and river water.

In every period and every time there are recommendations of how to live and some of these are valid for all places and all times of Earth while others are subject to change and evaluation.

Chapter One

Ayurveda ~ A loving science of how to take care of ourselves

Ayurveda guides us to become more loving and more aware of our lifestyles, diet and physical and mental exercises so as to attain perfect balance in spirit, body and mind. Ayurveda, written in Vedic Sanskrit, translates as "the science or knowledge of life". It believes in living a life of balance and harmony with our environment to prevent and to diminish disease. According to Ayurveda, a healthy lifestyle can be attained by:

- Preventive medicine whereby strengthening of the immune system is important.
- Treatment of disease after manifestation by herbs, syrups, tablets and various sorts of oils. It also recommends detoxification known as "Pancha Karma".
- To live a healthy lifestyle. This can be achieved by healthy diet, daily and seasonal disciplines.
- Ayurveda appreciates the uniqueness of each individual and strives to keep the individual constitution in balance.

Ayurveda originated about 5000 years ago from the ancient civilization of India as far back as the Indus Valley Civilization in the north-western part of the Indian subcontinent. It is one of the tenets of the Vedas, an aggregate of sacred texts and known to be the oldest of Sanskrit literature. The Vedas are a compilation of elaborate knowledge emerging from *Shruti* (meaning: what is heard) from the Divine and considered to be of "non human origin".

Ayurveda is part of the Vedas which were first presented in script by Srila Vyasadev, who one of the oldest seers from the Himalayas. The Vedas were written in Sanskrit. The Vedic scriptures elaborate on topics such as astrology, spirituality, governance, poetry, health and guidelines for healthy living. The Vedic texts are divided in to four main parts: Rig Veda (also known as Rik Veda), Sama Veda, Yajur Veda and Atharva Veda. Furthermore, there were two main schools of Ayurveda. One belonged to Atreya which was the academy of internists while the other belonged to Dhanvantari, and was the academy of surgeons. These two mainstreams eventually contributed to other scientific classifications of Ayurveda.

There were two main subsequent developments of Ayurveda which are still used as the basis for most of the Ayurvedic knowledge in present times: Sushruta and Charaka. The third important written scripture of Ayurveda is known as the Asthanga Hridaya. This is the shortened version of both Charaka and Sushruta. Originally, the vehicle of transmission of Ayurveda was done orally in the Sanskrit language which can be traced back between 2000 and 500 BC. The Sushruta first appeared during the 1st millennium BC and the Charaka is traced back to the 3rd century BC making Ayurveda the oldest existing healing system.

Culled from the divine, the ancient seers of the Indian subcontinent bestowed the Vedic scriptures to human kind. Ayurveda translates into the "knowledge of life". It is compiled from hymns from the Atharva-Veda and from the Rig-Veda. It denotes living a healthy lifestyle, in harmony with Mother Nature and recognises the internal microcosms within all living creatures as a crystal clear reflection of the outer realms of macrocosms. Prevention of disease is vital in Ayurveda as much as curing of any disease.

Ayurveda was gifted to human-kind by the Gods and deities to that are eternal and omnipresent up to date. Lord *Agni*, Shiva, *Vayu*, *Shakti* and *Prithvi* are but a few that whispered the key to sacred good health to the rishis. In the magnificent Vedic era, herbs, plants and fruits revealed their healing properties reminding us that we live in a heaven on Earth.

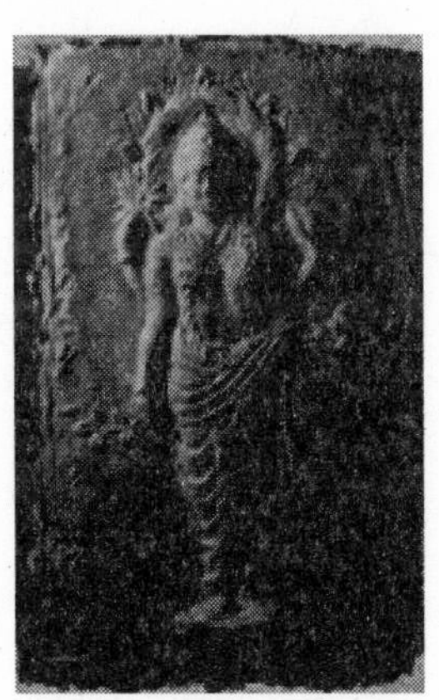

j jFigurejLordjDhanvatari

Ayurveda explains to us that the universe is composed of five elements: Ether, Air, Fire, Water and Earth and that these five elements exist in every living and non-living entity in different compositions, hence unique. When these five elements within human beings are "out of balance" to the natural state of healthy equilibrium then disease is formed. Ayurveda considers both the individual constitution as well as the constitution of the disease to carry the person back in to the harmony of good health. In simple words, excess of heat, i.e. *agni*, will cause illness in the human body related to heat, such as burn outs, ulcers or hyper acidity. This excess heat can be caused by lack of cold foods or cold environments, intake of excess alcohol or meat or peppers that increase heat in the human body. Ayurveda can be perceived as an art of living a healthy, happy and balanced lifestyle.

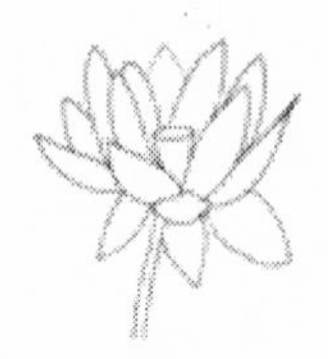

Om Namo Bhagavate
Maha Sudharshana
Vasudevaya Dhanvantaraye;
Amrutha Kalasa Hasthaaya
Sarva Bhaya Vinasaya
Sarva Roka Nivaranaya
Thri Lokya Pathaye
Thri Lokya Nithaye
Sri Maha Vishnu Swarupa
Sri Dhanvantri Swarupa
Sri Sri Sri
Aoushata Chakra Narayana Swaha

We prostate to the Lord, who is known as Sudarshana Vasudev Dhanvantari. He holds the Kalasha full of nectar of immortality. Lord Dhanvantri removes all fears and removes all diseases. He is the well wisher and the preserver of the three worlds. Dhanvantari is like Lord Vishnu, empowered to heal the Jiva souls. We pay reverence to the Lord of Ayurveda.

Chapter Two

Yoga

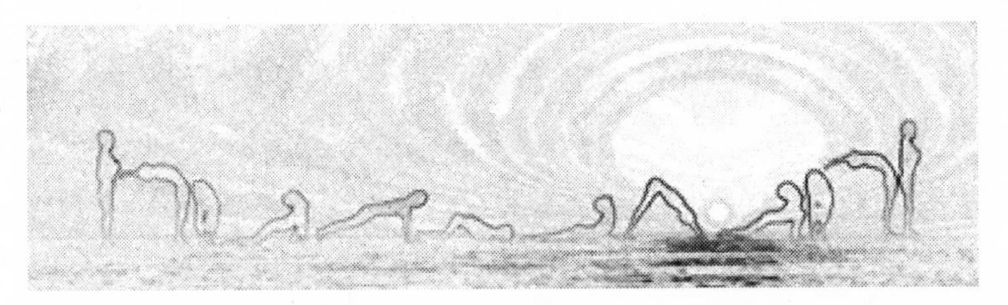

Yoga is an integral and essential aspect of Ayurveda. Yoga is derived from the Sanskrit word *yuj* which means "to join", "unity" or "oneness". In spiritual terms we can say that it means the oneness between the individual and undivided universal consciousness. Yoga is the balancing of body, mind and spirit. There are many branches of *yoga*: *raja*, *hatha*, *jnana*, *karma*, *bhakti*, *mantra*, *kundalini* and *laya* and more. Yoga can be defined as the union between limited self (*jiva*) and the cosmic self (*atman*). In a way, there is no separation between the two, yet for there to be an aim of the union, there must be a separation. The aim as such, of yoga, is not to unite us with anything rather to help us realize our Higher Self. Yoga helps us transcend our everyday normal life or individual consciousness unto our true inner nature.

The origin of yoga can be traced in ancient India as well as in other parts of the world more than ten thousand years ago. Many deities resembling Lord Shiva and Parvati performing various *asanas* and practices of meditation have been found in archaeological excavations made in the Indus Valley at Harappa and at Mohenjo-Daro, now known as modern Pakistan. These ruins were once a dwelling place of people who lived in the pre-Vedic age before the Aryan civilization flourished in the Indian subcontinent. Yoga arose at the start of the human civilization as when man first realized his spiritual potential and strived to evolve techniques to develop it.

The first books to refer to yoga were the ancient Tantras and later the Vedas which were written around the time that the Indus Valley culture was flourishing. Yoga was presented symbolically until it first took a more definable shape in the Upanishads and finally collectively formed the *Vedanta*. Sage Patanjali finally codified the first definitive, unified and comprehensive system of yoga in his Yoga Sutras. He laid down the essential foundations of yoga. Today yoga has succeeded as an alternative form of therapy in diseases like asthma, diabetes, blood pressure, arthritis, digestive disorders and many more ailments. Research has also shown positive results on HIV as well as for nervous and endocrine system disorders. For most people, however, yoga is simply a means to maintain health and well-being in the modern day stressful world. Yoga, however, need not just be seen as a handy physical exercise. It is rather a means that embraces both inner and outer realities and a way of life that cannot just be understood intellectually. From the physical body, yoga moves unto the physical and emotional body and can aid in recovering from phobias, psychosomatic ailments and neuroses from stresses in life. Yoga might not provide a cure for life's problems but it certainly does provide a proven method for coping with it.

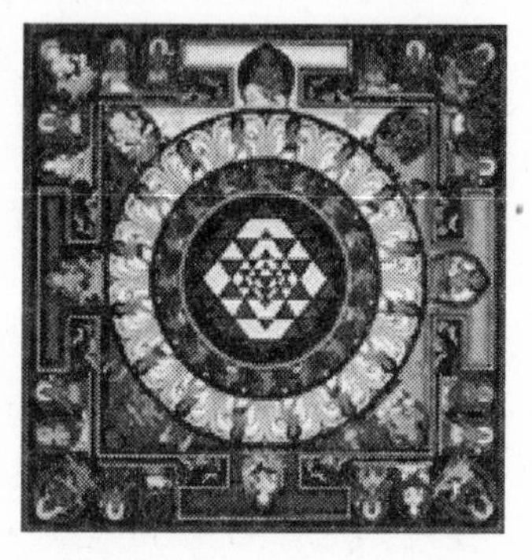

j jFigurejYantrajofjVedicjSymbols

The fundamental yogic practices include asanas, postures; pranayamas, breathing techniques; mudras, positions or gestures which represent the psyche; bandhas, locks for channelling energy; and shatkarmas, cleansing practices. The ideal practices that complement Ayurveda are *asanas*, *pranayamas* and *mantra* chanting.

In Sanskrit, *asana* means "pose". It denotes being in steady or comfortable postures. It is believed that *asanas* were physical exercises as they are known to have a profound influence on the body. At the same time, and as the Vedas tell us, each person is made of body, mind and consciousness, and practising of *asanas* aims at harmonizing all these three aspects.

It is written in the ancient text on yoga, Hatha Yoga Pradipika, that 'Life is a period between one breath and the next; a person who only half breathes, only half lives. He, who breathes correctly, acquires control of the whole being." The ancient yogis were fully aware of the importance of breath. Simply put, if there is no breath, then there is no life. Pranayama refers to breathing. In yoga, it is said that each person has a fixed number of breaths allocated to him in one lifetime. Hence, if one breathes slowly one will live longer and if one breathes rapidly than one is using up the allocated number of breaths faster resulting in decreasing one's life-span. A fast breathing rate is also associated with tension, fear, worry which in turn leads to bad health and unhappiness. Conversely, if a person breathes slowly as well as deeply the lungs are filled to a greater depth. This helps to remove stagnant air that is also filled with germs. Naturally, shallow breathing connected with fast breathing does not allow pure oxygenated blood to purify the entire body. In consequence, mental and physical ailments are formed. In ancient times, the human race was more receptive to the rhythms of nature which include the process of breathing.

In a way, modern materialistic life with its technosphere has distracted us from harmonious breathing.

The Sanskrit word *mudra* can be translated in to "attitude" or "gesture". While some involve the entire body, most are performed with the hands and fingers. *Mudras* can be psychic, emotional, devotional or aesthetic; hence, each *mudra* has its own specific effect on the practitioner.

Another small but important group of yogic practices are *bandhas*. The Sanskrit word *bandha* means 'to hold' or "to lock" which is precisely the action necessary to perform these practices. Specific parts of the body are gently but tightly contacted and tightened. Traditional yogic texts speak of ganthis, or psychic blocks and mental problems which prevent a person from properly experiencing higher states of awareness. These *ganthis* are located in the pelvis, heart and centre of the head. *Bandhas* are very effective in breaking open or removing these blocks either temporarily or permanently. Although, *bandhas* have a direct influence on the psychic body or else pranic body and not the physical or mental body, it is important to realize that these are interrelated.

Bandhas are essential in regulating proper flow of prana, or vital force, throughout the body as well as to prevent the *prana* from dissipating. The three important *bandhas* are the *Jalandhara bandha*, *Uddiyana bandha* and *Mula bandha.*

The *Jalandhara bandha* regulates the flow of *prana* and blood to the heart, the glands in the neck and head and the brain. If *pranayama* is performed without the *Jalandhara bandha* then pressure might be felt in the heart, behind the eyeballs and the ear cavities and the head can feel dizzy. This *bandha* is performed by contracting the neck and the throat while the chin is made to rest on the chest in the notch between the collar-bones and at the top of the breast-bone.

The *Uddiyana bandha* is known to be one of the best of the *bandhas* and promotes longetivity or helps make a person young again. The process of *Uddiyana bandha* is to lift the diaphragm high up the thorax and to pull in the abdominal organs against the back towards the spine. It exercises the diaphragm and the abdominal organs. The cavity created by the lift of the diaphragm gives a gentle massage to the muscles of the heart, thereby toning it.

The *Mula bandha* is the region between the anus and the scrotum. By contracting the region, the *prana* in the lower abdomen whose course is downwards (apana vayu) is made to flow up and unite with the main *prana* which has its seat in the region of its chest. *Mula bandha* should first be attempted by retention of breath after inhalation. The region of the lower abdomen between the navel and the anus is contracted towards the diaphragm.

In the *Uddiyana Bandha,* the entire region from the anus to the diagram up to the sternum is pulled back towards the spine and lifted up. But in *Mula Bandha,* the whole lower abdominal area between the anus and the navel is contracted, pulled back to the spine and lifted up towards the diaphragm.

The practice of yoga is a reflection of our fundamental attitudes towards life and their physical counterparts in the body. Yoga, though an ancient science, evolved over thousands of years dealing with the physical, moral, mental and spiritual well-being of man as a whole. Today, we have the option of practising yoga in several places or else taking some time at home on a daily regular or weekly irregular basis for yogic exercises for our well-being.

Chapter Three

Today's Ayurveda

Nowadays, Ayurveda is commonly perceived as an alternative or complementary form of healing. It is often compared with Traditional Chinese Medicine or else is well-known for its massage therapies. Only few might realize it to be a vast holistic system of medicine. In 1970s, the Indian government decided on standardizing Ayurvedic education with qualifications and accreditations and to support in research. Outside India, Ayurvedic scholars have gained in recognition in the Western world by increasing their research and development and by creating educational systems. This has helped in reviving Ayurveda and making it of benefit globally. Ayurvedic practitioners require a license to practice in the United States of America. The Gujarat Ayurveda University has also signed a Memorandum of Understanding (MoU) with nine Ayurvedic institutes functioning in Japan, Australia, the Netherlands, Italy, Argentina, and Germany to coordinate and facilitate the globalization of Ayurveda through academic collaboration. Prior to this, the Medical (*Ayu*) Institute of Russia had also signed the MoU with the government of India, in which the Gujarat Ayurved University is also one of the implementing authorities. Today, scientific research continues on Ayurvedic treatments. Ayurveda is also recognized by the World Health Organisation (WHO) as part of traditional medicine upon which a significant number of persons depend on very successfully.

Ideally, Ayurveda encompasses 'a science of life' that could take beyond a lifetime to grasp. At the same time, when one takes a closer look at the guidelines described in the Vedic texts, they are profoundly simple. The guidelines only need to be synchronized to become applicable to other parts of the world, beyond the Indian subcontinent where Ayurveda was originally conceived. Avocados or Kiwis, for instance, do not grow in India, hence, if we were to follow Ayurveda, should we stop eating avocados and kiwis? Rather, it is logical to know the properties of these fruits in relation to bodily humours. Similarly, India is known to have six seasons, including a rainy season with recommendations of an Ayurvedic seasonal lifestyle known as "Rtucharya", but is that applicable in the Sahara Desert as well? It is therefore clear that the original guidelines need continuous revision. In his book, "The Yoga of Herbs", David Frawley suggests that plants be approached for their healing properties in respect of their tastes which are an important aspect in Ayurveda. Sweet and sour tastes, for instance, are said to be incompatible in Ayurveda as they produce toxins. Ayurveda helps us reawaken our innate wisdom no matter whom we are or where we are.

In our world today, we often live alienated from nature because we are connected to technology and machines to a large degree. We rely on machines for transportation, use computers or microwaves to warm up our meals. There is a lot of indifference and a sense of apathy in how people can feel in cosmopolitan cities and individualistic societies. People are often in a hurry to solve never-ending problems. We also have to cope with new diseases, eating genetically manipulated foods or breathing toxic wastes from factories of large multi-nationals. People have become mechanized in their lifestyles and victims to haste. Most importantly, many of us have forgotten to relax and to appreciate the music of silence. At the same time ultimately, we all seek true happiness and well-being.

The purpose of Ayurveda is not only to cure the diseases we suffer from but also to prevent diseases and to live a happy lifestyle. This is well outlined in recommendations made for daily, seasonal and ethical guidelines. If we are able to embrace even just a few of these recommendations we shall undoubtedly relish a healthy and joyful life. This also enables us to have clarity and peace of mind with virtuous qualities such as patience, gratitude, forgiveness, compassion, humour and an overall positive outlook unto life. Following Ayurveda gives a mental stability that works on all levels and as we know many dis-eases are now proven to be psychosomatic.

Today's Ayurveda is as precious as when culled from the Divine 5000 years ago. It reminds us of our innate supreme nature, a nature that is lovable and caring inside-out. Ayurveda believes in a micro- and macro-cosmos. It states that everything outside is merely a reflection of what is inside each and every one of us. It encourages the practice of Ayurvedic sadhanas, spiritual practices, just so that we can awaken cosmic memory and be at peace and harmony with Mother Nature as well. *Sadhanas* can include walking bare feet on sand or grass, preparing meals in love and harmony and organic gardening. Surely, it is worth being aware and respecting that our bodies need food devoid of insecticides and poisons or else food that are neither too little nor too much for our needs? Ayurveda does not ask us to perform miracles nor to live up to impossible and outdated expectations but simply to awaken to our full potentials. Luckily science is catching up and acknowledging the holistic and traditional medicines and ways of life such as Ayurveda.

Chapter Four

"Dincharya"

Dincharya in Ayurvedic texts refers to daily guidelines for personal hygiene. Different times of the day have their own doshic (*vata* (ether+air), *pitta* (fire) and *kapha* (water and earth)) peaks in relation to the earth's dynamic relationship to both the sun and the moon. This is shown in table below:

SEVEN DAILY CYCLES OF THE *DOSHAS*

	VATA	*PITTA*	*KAPHA*
DAWN	Dominant	Neutral	Accumulating
MORNING	Lessening	Accumul ating	Dominant
MID-DAY	Neutral	Dominant	Lessening
AFTERNOON	Accumulating	Lessening	Neutral
DUSK	Dominant	Neutral	Accumulating
EARLY EVENING	Lessening	Accumulating	Dominant
MIDNIGHT	Neutral	Dominant	Lessening

VATA	Dominant 2:00 – 6:00 am & pm
PITTA	Dominant 10:00 – 2:00 am & pm
KAPHA	Dominant 6:00 – 10:00 am & pm

It is recommended that people should awaken before sunrise and should then cater to the natural excretory urges known as *malas*. These include stool and urine of course. All the excretory orifices can best be cleansed with water. Doing some light exercise after this, especially in the form of yoga every morning is healthy. Exercise can include some breathing exercises as well in the form of *pranayama*, some *mantra* chanting and some *vipassana* meditation. If desired, *bandhas* can also be practised. Although, it would be best to devote at least 30 minutes to an hour to daily yoga practice, many are unable to manage this in our modern times. As such, it might be best to compromise disciplining oneself into doing 15-30 minutes daily morning yoga practice rather than no exercise at all. One can begin with sitting in a comfortable position with loose clothing and by bringing one's awareness to one's breathing and following the flow of the in and out-coming breath in accordance to the belly going out and in respectfully. When ready, the Gayatri mantra may optionally be chanted thrice:

"Om bhur bhuva svaha, tatsaviture vareniyam,
bhargo devasya dhimahi, dhio yo na pracho dayat"

This beautiful Gayatri is considered to be one of the holiest verses of the Vedas as Gayatri is the Mother of the Vedas. A well-related interpretation of the Gayatri *mantra* is by Sir William Jones , a Welsh philologist particularly known for his proposition of the existence of a relationship among Indo-European languages and he has also been a student of ancient India:

"Let us adore the supremacy of that Divine Sun, the God head, who illuminates all, who recreates all, from whom all proceed, to whom all must return, whom we invoke to direct our understanding aright in our progress towards his holy seat."

After chanting of the Gayatri mantra thrice, one may begin with pranayamic breathing for a couple of minutes. The commonest one is the alternative nostril breathing known as Nadi Shodhana Pranayama. This is done by:

1) Closing the right nostril with the right thumb and breathing in deeply from the left nostril while the belly rises. Then exhaling from the right nostril by closing the right nostril with the index finger twice the time of inhalation and allowing the belly to fall.

2) Then once again, inhaling from the same right nostril while the index finger keeps the left nostril closed and allowing the belly to rise. Then again to close the right nostril with the right thumb and exhaling double the amount of time from the left nostril.

This practice is highly beneficial to everyone as it cleanses the solar and lunar channels and makes the mind silent and alert. It also removes excess *kapha* from the body.

The Nadi Shodhana Pranayama can best be followed by *Kappalabhati.*

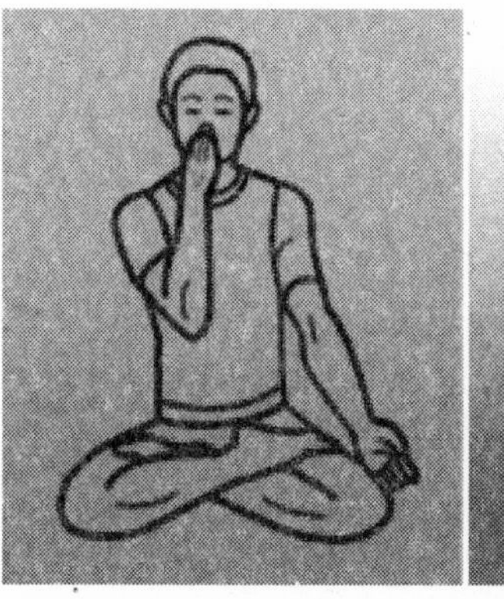
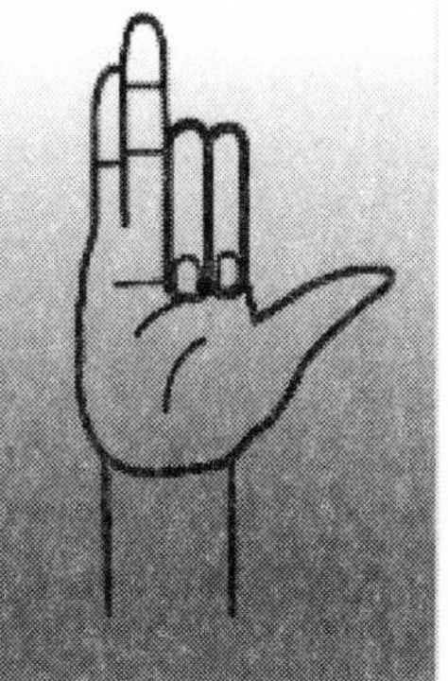

The *Kappalabhati* is performed by first sitting in a comfortable position and then inhaling deeply through both nostrils, expanding the abdomen and then exhaling with the forceful contraction of abdominal muscles. (The abdomen should be pulled in by quickly contracting the abdominal muscles and exhaling through the nose). The air is pushed out of the lungs by the subsequent contraction of the diaphragm. Inhaling should be effortless, simply allowing the body to do what it does best. The focus should be on exhalation. It is important not to hold your breath during these exercises; it is the method of breathing that is important.

Try starting off with 10 to 15 inhalations/exhalations (we can call this a round). After one round relax and breath (inhale and exhale) deeply a few times, then start another round. Three rounds are sufficient (especially for beginners).

Some of the many benefits from practising *Kappalabhati* are the cleansing of the lungs and respiratory system. Improved digestion, natural strengthening and toning of the abdominal muscles and energizing of the mind. As with most types of *pranayama*, precautions should be made if one suffers from any form of heart disease or hypertension.

After the *Kappalabhati*, one can begin with some warm up exercises and some *asanas*. One can begin by rotating the head thrice clockwise and then anti-clockwise. Then the shoulders are to be raised thrice and made to fall thrice. Then to rotate the hands thrice clockwise and then anti-clockwise. Finally, the feet can be rotated thrice from the ankles, also thrice clockwise and anti-clockwise.

Head rolls

1. Inhale: sit upright in a comfortable seated position, with your arms and shoulders relaxed. Exhale: lower your chin down toward your sternum.
2. Inhale: gently roll your head up and to the side to look over your left shoulder. Make the movement as soft and fluid as possible.
3. Continue to roll your head up on the inhalation to look up toward the ceiling. Make sure that your shoulder blades are relaxed down your back.
4. Exhale: slowly drop your head to the opposite side to look over your right shoulder. Continue to roll your head down and back to the first position.

Repeat the exercise twice in one direction and twice in the opposite direction. If you find some discomfort in your neck, rest in that position briefly and breathe into the area to release the tension.

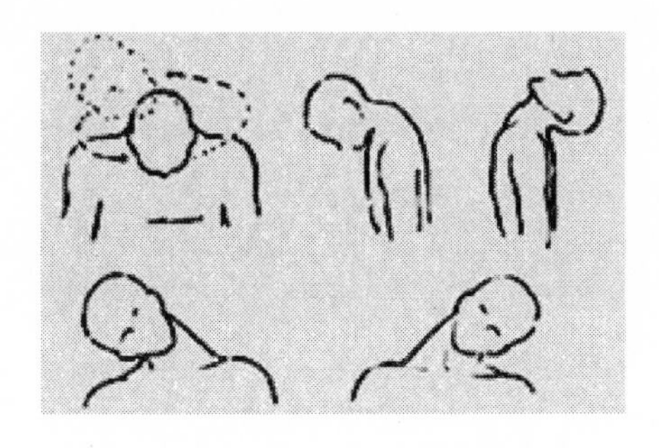

Sitting side stretch

1. Sit upright in a comfortable cross-legged position. Place your right hand on the mat a few cm from your right hip with your fingers pointing toward the end of the mat.
2. Rotate your left arm until your palm is facing the ceiling.

Inhale: lift your left arm up and over your head to the right, so that you feel the stretch along the entire left side of your body.

Exhale: keep your left 'sit' bones (in your buttocks) firmly grounded on the floor as you stay in the stretch.

Breath: hold the pose for eight or more breaths. Release the pose and repeat on the other side.

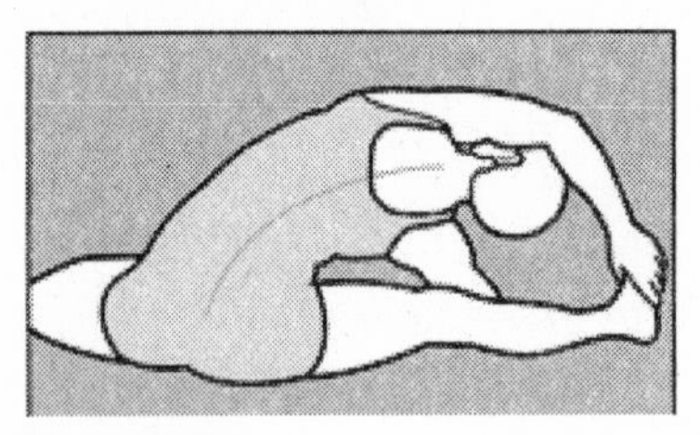

Sitting forward stretch

1. Sit on the ground. Place the left heel pressing hard near the left groin. Keep the right leg stretched and straight. Hold the right foot with the hands. Exhale and draw the stomach in.
2. Lower the head slowly as shown in the figure. Place the forehead and the chin on the knee. Remain in this position for five to ten seconds.

Breath: Release the pose and inhale and repeat on the other side.

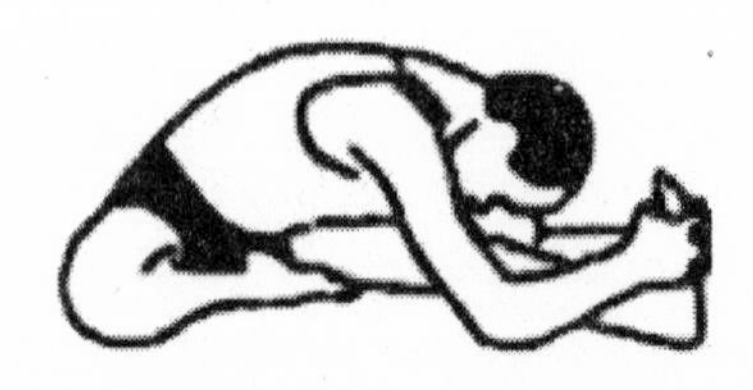

One knee to chest

1. Lie flat on your back on the mat, with your feet together. Raise your right leg and then bend your knee. Clasp both your hands firmly around your shin, just below the knee.
2. Inhale: take a deep breath in. Exhale: hug your bent leg close to your chest. Keep your straight leg strong by pushing in to your left heel. Try to push your tailbone (coccyx) down toward the floor. Relax your head and neck and make sure there is no tension in your jaw.

Breath: Keep breathing evenly for eight or more breaths. Release the pose and repeat on the other side.

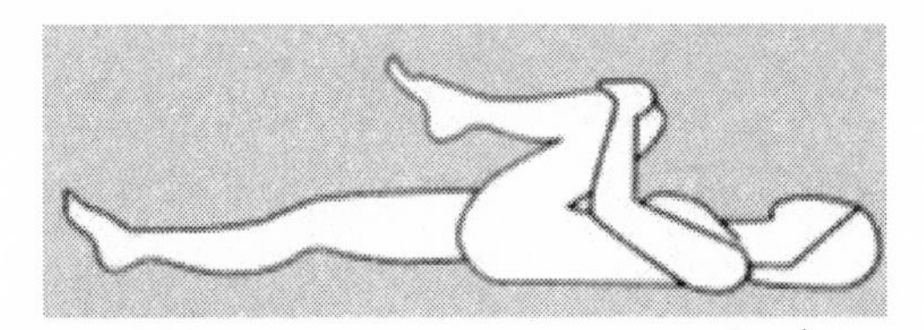

One knee to the side

1. Inhale: Lie flat on your back with your feet together. Raise your left leg and bend your knee. Hold your leg just below the knee with your left hand.
2. Exhale: Draw your knee close to your chest and then drop your knee out to the left side, rotating it from the hip. Keep your right leg strong by pushing in to your heel and drawing your toes toward you.

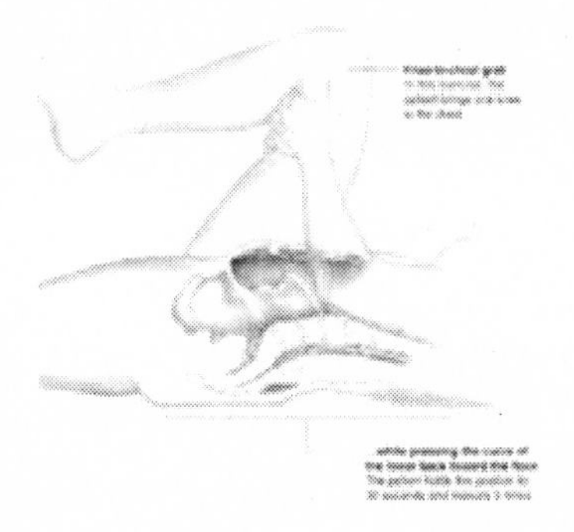

Breath: Keep breathing evenly for eight or more breaths. Release the pose and repeat on the other side.

Head to knees forward bend

1. Sit with both legs extended straight in front of you.
2. Make sure the legs are parallel and feet pointing straight up.
3. Inhale: Reach forward with your hands and hold onto your legs as low as possible without bending the knees.
4. If you can hold your toes that is great, if not, arch them back towards you while holding your shins, knees or thighs. This will ensure you are stretching the calves and nerves.
5. As you reach towards your feet, ensure you are bending from the waist and try to keep the back as straight as possible. Exhale and try to bring the forehead to the knees if possible.

Breath: hold the pose for five to six breaths. Inhale and release the pose returning to original position.

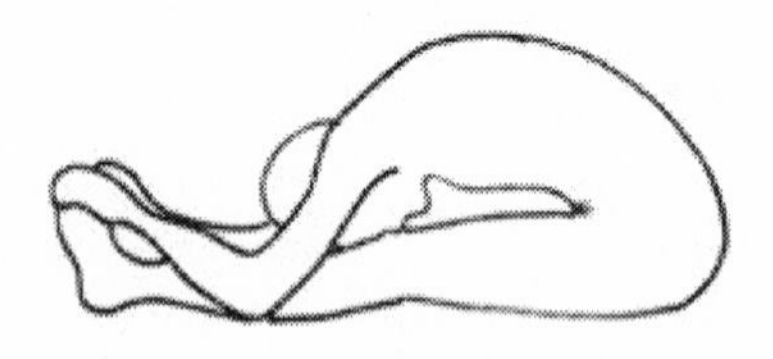

Cat stretch

1. Move from a kneeling position on the mat to come up on all fours. Place your hands directly under your shoulders with your middle fingers pointing forward. Place your knees in line with your hips a few cm apart, with your toes pointing backwards.
2. Inhale: Lift your tailbone (coccyx) and sacrum toward the ceiling, making your lower back concave, until your head lifts naturally toward the ceiling.
3. Exhale: Tuck your tail under and arch your back toward the ceiling, allowing the action in the lower back to initiate the movement through the upper spine. Tuck your head in,

pointing your chin toward the sternum. Repeat up to ten times in slow rhythmic motions in time with your breathing.

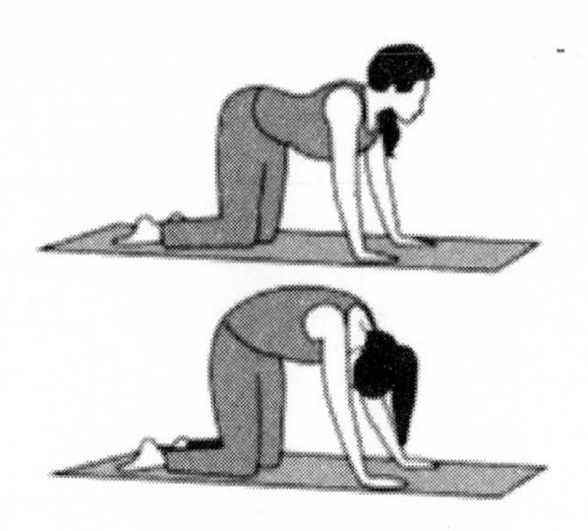

Lunge

1. Kneel with your thighs parallel. Bend your left leg and position it on the floor in front of you so that it forms a right angle. Keep your spine straight and place a hand on top of your left knee.
2. With both hands on your left knee, lunge forward by increasing the bend in your left knee. Tuck your tailbone under and drop your right thigh and groin towards the floor. Keep your head and chest lifted.

Breath: Keep breathing evenly for eight or more breaths. Release the pose and repeat on the other side.

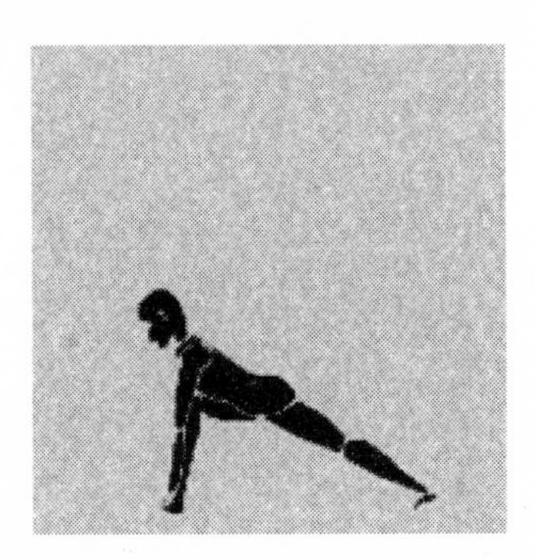

Surya Namaskar – Sun Salutation

Surya namaskar is supreme for its totality in exercise. It is a dynamic series of fourteen *asanas* that are linked together with the breath. The flow of each *asana* helps to create heat in the body, which limbers up the spine and tones the joints, muscles, and internal organs. The sun salutation series regulates the solar plexus or pingala nadi which conducts vitality and energy through the body.

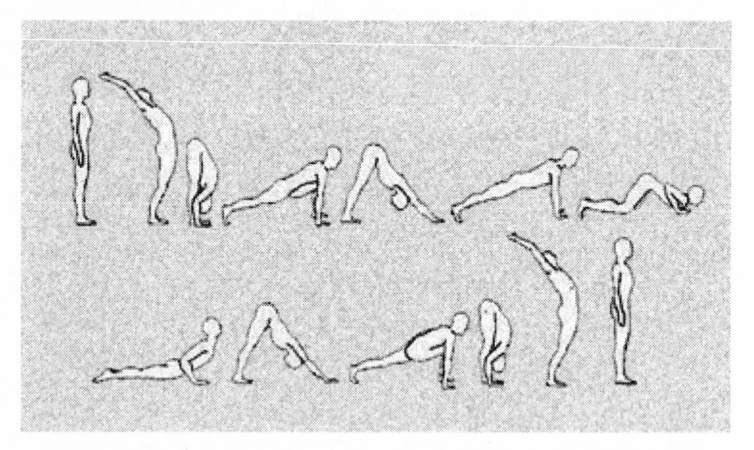

1. Stand upright in tadasana pose (see picture) at the front of the mat with your feet together, and your hands together in – Namaste position.
2. Inhale: stretch your arms up, interlock your hands and point upward with you index fingers so that your feel the stretch evenly along both sides of your body. Look up towards your thumbs, without tipping your head too far back.
3. Lift your chest toward the ceiling to open your heart centre. Do not strain your lower back.
4. Exhale: Bend forward from your hips, keeping your back and knees straight. Relax your head down toward your knees and put your hands on the mat next to your feet. If your hands do not quite touch the floor then bend your knees.

5. Inhale: stretch your left leg out behind you and drop your left knee to the floor. Move your chest forward and look up.
6. Come up onto your toes and take your right foot back in line with your left. Lower your buttocks so that your back is in one inclined plane, with your head in line with your spine.

   Breath: Keep holding the breath.
7. Exhale: Bend your knees to the floor and lower your chest to the floor between your bent arms and hands, leaving your pelvis raised. Place your chin on the floor.
8. Inhale: Tuck your tailbone under and slide your body weight forward. Press down in to the palms of your hands and stretch out your spine, lifting up your head, neck, and chest. Look up toward the ceiling, but make sure your pelvis is still on the floor.
9. Exhale: Push into your hands, raise your buttocks up in to the air and back so that your body forms a triangle. Relax the crown of your head toward the floor and release your neck. Keep lengthening the spine and press your heels toward the floor.
10. Inhale: Lift your left leg forward, in line with your hands. Bend your right knee and release your pelvis down.
11. Lift your chest forward, lengthen the spine, and look up.
12. Exhale: Come into forward bend by bringing your right foot forward to line up with your left foot. Lift up your thighs and straighten through the backs of your legs. Relax your head down toward your knees.
13. Inhale: Flatten your back, reach up, and out until you are back at step 3.
14. Release the stretch and return to step 2.

15. Exhale: Bring your hands back down in front of your chest. Inhale: Repeat this cycle, taking your right leg back first to complete one full round of surya namaskar.

In yoga, the sun symbolizes spiritual consciousness and, in ancient times, was worshipped on a daily basis. The dynamic group of *asanas*, belonging to the surya namaskar, is an effective way of loosening up, stretching, massaging and toning all the joints, muscles and internal organs of the body. Surya namaskar is a complete sadhana, spiritual practice, in itself for it includes *asana*, *pranayama*, *mantra* and also meditation techniques. Inevitably, regular practice of surya namaskar leads to a balanced system at both mental and physical levels. It is an excellent group of *asanas* with which to begin the morning.

After yoga, one can begin with a cleansing routine of the body. The person should wash his or her hands and mouth followed by brushing of teeth. Toothpaste did not exist in ancient times but herbal toothpastes in our present times are best to use. Otherwise, if desired and attainable, the ancient tradition can be kept by brushing with frayed twigs of the Neem tree (Azadirachta indicahi, syn. Melia azadirachta L., Antelaea azadirachta (L.) Adelb.) or else The Miswak (miswaak, siwak) makes a good natural toothbrush which is made from the twigs of the Salvadora persica tree, also known as the Arak tree or the Peelu tree. Other tree types that can be used are the olive, walnut, and any other such trees with bitter roots. Liquorice root (Glycyrrhiza glabra) can also be used which is sweet and salty in taste. In Africa, frayed twigs from the Salvadore Persica trees can be used.

Tongue scraping is also typical of a standard Ayurvedic morning regime. It is said that this releases repressed emotions or toxins, known as Ama in Sanskrit, which appear as a whitish or yellow layer on the tongue. Curved U-shaped metal strips or spoons can be used, preferably made of gold, silver, copper, tin or brass. Tongue –scraping is followed by gargling, best done with some drops of sesame oil in water as recommended in Ayurveda. It said to prevent loosening of teeth, prevention of a dry throat or mouth and it triggers one's appetite. It also improves on one's voice. Eye washes with luke warm water or even eye drops are recommended to improve vision and to avoid eye disorders or even migraines. This also refreshes the mind. Adding some drops of sesame oil into clean water and using them as eye drops is also part of the Ayurvedic regime. Oiling of ears also helps in migraines as well as cleansing of ears and prevention of ear ailments.

The next steps of the *dincharya* are to oil the head or body. Sesame oil is again the best oil that can be used for all constitutions as it is a neutral as well as a sattvic or pure oil. *Sattva* in Sanskrit stands for that which is pure. Other oils are Thripaladi oil, which includes a combination of three Ayurvedic fruits - Amalaki, Bibhitaki, Haritaki and Dhanwantari oil made of the herbs Neem and Shatavari.

A jar or bottle of oil can best be kept in one's bathroom for anointing of the body before the shower. Oiling maintains skin lustre and also provides nourishment to the skin, it being one of the most important organs of the body. Oiling also helps in keeping the *doshas* in balance thereby helping in prevention of diseases. Finally, bathing or showering can be done without using chemical soaps. In fact it is best to use no soap rather than to use soaps with chemicals. Natural soaps or aroma oils can best be used. Some oils that can be used in the bath in accordance to *doshas* are mentioned in the following tables:

Doshas	**Base Oil**
Vata	Sesame
Pitta	Coconut or sunflower
Kapha	Canola or mustard
Doshas	Aroma Oils
Vata	Musk, Basil, Camphor, Rose, Cinnamon or Sandalwood
Pitta	Rose, Sandalwood, Lotus, Lily, Lavender or Iris
Kapha	Cinnamon, musk, sage, cedar or myrrh

Ayurveda recommends in never holding back on natural urges like sneezing or else wishing to go to the bathroom. It recommends wearing clothes of natural fibre and those that are clean. Nowadays, there are also many washing detergents available without chemicals and without animal testing. It is said in the *Charaka* that beautiful clothes enhance one's charm and life span, give pleasure and make it enjoyable to be around others. Using incense perfumes, such as aroma therapy oils, scented soap and flowers also promote longevity, charm, strength and nourishment. They also enhance pleasing manners and similar to the clothing remove inauspiciousness. Wearing ornaments related to gem therapy promote wealth, auspiciousness, longevity, happiness and ojas, our life giving essence. Cutting hair, nails, beard/moustache is life-promoting, beautifies and cleans. Sunrise is a wonderful time to have the eyes in the direction of the first rays of sunlight (though not looking directly in to the sun for too long). This exercise improves one's vision and vitality. It is important to receive sunlight daily, when possible. Naturally, taking in sunlight in the winter is more difficult because there is simply less sunlight. Sunlight is the best source of vitamins D4 and D5. In any case it is best to avoid remaining in the dark for long periods of time, even if it means foregoing some of those candle-light atmospheres in the dark winter months of some parts of the world. Ayurveda also recommends that it is important to find livelihood that is not contradictory to one's dharma (God-given talents). Finally, Ayurveda asks of us to practice sadhanas (meditation or spiritual practices) preferably according to the instructions of one's *guru* (spiritual teacher) if one has a guru of course. In Ayurveda, insights into the science of mind and body were seen as inter-dependent and a complete system of psychological healing and virtuous conduct, thus meditation plays a key aspect to our well-being.

Chapter Five

"ऋतुcharya ...... Rtucharya"

Mother Nature governs laws in which similar is homologous and hence enriches the similar whilst dissimilar is heterologous and hence it depletes. This is known as samanya and visesa in Sanskrit. Ayurveda guides us to manage our *doshas* in accordance to the changes of seasons by adapting our lifestyles and diet. This is the practice of Rtucharya. Ayurveda especially cautions us to pay some extra attention to maintaining equilibrium of our *doshas* during transitional periods between two seasons when disease most commonly might occur.

Generally, a season can be described by changes in weather during the course of the year. Seasons are a result of the Earth's orbit around the sun and the tilt of its own axis relative to plane of revolution. The latter means the planet's rotational axis in relation to its orbital plane. During the months of June, July and August, the Earth's northern hemisphere is exposed to more direct sunlight because the northern hemisphere then faces the sun as the Earth tilts. The same is true for the southern hemisphere in the months of December, January, and February. As is common knowledge, there are usually four seasons defined in temperate and polar regions: spring, summer, autumn, winter. In sub tropical and tropical regions, however, where it is more common to have a lot of precipitation there is also the rainy (or monsoon) season and in some parts of the world seasons are also defined in accordance to hurricane season, tornado season and wildfire season.

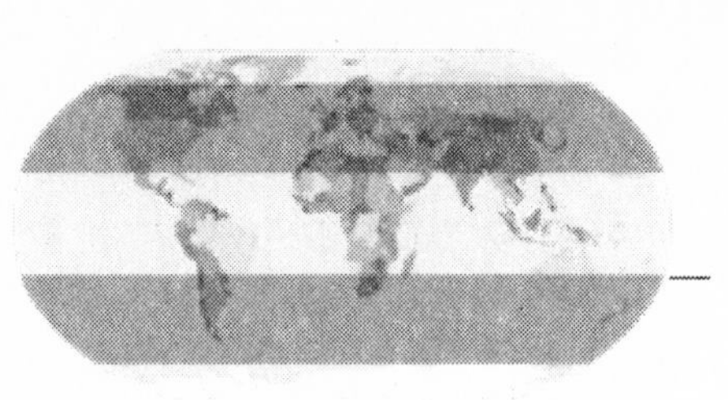

j jFigurejjWorldjMapjtemperatejzonesjhighj lightedjinjred

Since the Vedic period unto this day and age, India recognizes six seasons: pre-winter, winter, spring, summer, monsoon and autumn. Ayurveda embraces the natural appearance of *doshas* in these six seasons as follows in the table:

	Accumulation	**Aggravation**	**Alleviation**
VATA	Summer	Rainy season (early autumn), late winter	Autumn
PITTA	Rainy season	Autumn, Rainy season (early autumn)	Early winter
KAPHA	Early winter	Spring, Rainy season (early autumn)	Summer

From late winter unto spring and summer, the absorbing effects of the sun and wind progressively rise until their culmination in mid-June. The tastes bitter, astringent and pungent are enhanced during this northerly phase of the sun and they share a constricting and absorbent nature so when used in food can further deplete an organism.

The sun then commences its southward movement across the earth to the rainy season, autumn and early winter. The heat of the sun decreases progressively until its culmination in mid-November. During this period, the sun and the wind are restrained in the clouds and rains triggering a period of cool release. The remaining three tastes sweet, sour and salty are greatly enhanced and contribute to bulk and vigour when consumed by an organism.

As mentioned earlier, our bodies are particularly vulnerable during the junction of seasons, known as rtusandhi, in Sanskrit and we are advised to make extra efforts during the last seven days of the previous season and the first seven days of the new season. It is a time that we are most susceptible to being unwell.

In the region in and around to the Netherlands, four seasons are marked. However, the climate fluctuates considerably so that there might be rainfall on some mornings in some summer months with temperatures declining and then suddenly rising when the sun offers its warmth in the afternoon, all in a small stretch of time. It is best to consider these changes when following the guidelines of rtucharya while the general appearances of *doshas* in this region are:

	Accumulation	**Aggravation**	**Alleviation**
VATA	Autumn	Autumn	Summer
PITTA	Spring	Summer	Autumn
KAPHA	Autumn	Winter	Spring

The predominance of the six tastes in accordance to the seasons remains unchanged.

Vedic and Ayurvedic literature generally regard 'time' or "kala" in Sanskrit as being responsible for creating, maintaining, and destroying. Different intervals in time have unique creative values. Time is also defined by solar and lunar perspectives. Days and seasons as solar references and lunar phases relate to rites, rituals, planting and harvest times. It is beneficial to regard dincharya and rtucharya in our lives as much as possible for our well-being. Dincharya and rtucharya are also important in Pancha Karma treatment. The term 'Pancha Karma' refers to the five main practices used to cleanse the body of its excess bodily humours or *doshas.* It is a highly beneficial therapy in Ayurveda. Dincharya is particularly an important post Pancha Karma treatment while *rtucharya* is very beneficial during the Pancha Karma treatment. In any case, many of the din charya recommendations are quite feasible and one can make a gradual transition to a better daily lifestyle.

Chapter Six

Diet

'All the world seeks food. It is the life source of all beings. Clarity, longetivity, intelligence, happiness, contentment, strength and knowledge are all rooted in food'

- Charaka

Diet is essential in Ayurveda. While it is always considered in every ayurvedic therapy, its proper application can sometimes even be the remedy itself. The five main considerations of ayurvedic dietetics are the quantity one eats, the time and season the food is taken, mood during preparation and cooking, food habits and constitution of the person who is to eat the food as well as the climate of the particular day.

Charaka Samhita identifies the first foods on Mother Earth as rice, barley, mung beans, amalaki (Indian gooseberry) fruit, rain water, rock salt, honey, milk and ghee. These are considered to be wholesome foods and beneficial to us in many ways. Naturally, people must consider their allergic susceptibility to these foods with an Ayurvedic doctor or practitioner in case any of these foods feel inappropriate. Intake of water is also important in Ayurveda. Water is the most important element on earth as well as for the human body. There is about 60% water in adult males and 55% in adult females.

According to Ayurveda, 'food' is sacred and is referred to as God itself in the Taittiriya Upanishad and presented as such not only in respect to the nutritional aspect. The rishis conveyed to us that whilst eating we are in communion with God or the universe whilst we process foods we are awakening our cognitive memories. We tend to become distracted by our busy minds or activities and forget the spiritual vastness and oneness that we truly are. The Vedic texts also tell us that the single most auspicious animal is the cow and food derived from the cow. Naturally, these days we must strive to consume plants and animals that have lived a healthy life. In the Vedas, which preceded Ayurveda, it is maintained that human food is primarily of plant origin. Milk, particularly cow milk is considered to be wholesome and most pure or sattvic for us.

Ayurveda also tells us that foods can have three qualities or attributes: *Sattvic*, *Rajasic*, and *Tamasic*. These are called gunas in Sanskrit. In fact, each and every living species is of varying combinations of these three gunas. *Sattva* denotes happiness, peace and calm, bliss, clarity and quiet of the mind. *Sattvic* foods are calm inducing and offer a sense of fulfilment irrespective of our actions in the sense that we approach whatever we do in balance rather than being too goal orientated. Foods that nourish us with *sattva guna* are good quality milk, ghee, wheat, and fruits or dried foods that are sweet and cooling. Mung daal and Basmati rice are particularly *Sattvic* in nature as well as large leafy vegetables. *Sattvic* herbs include basil, cardamom, cinnamon, coriander, cumin, fennel, fenugreek and turmeric. Hot and pungent spices like garlic, ginger or pepper are not *Sattvic*.

"We are what we eat" is still not an uncommon expression in our times and suggests that we consider what foods we consume. Ayurveda acknowledges that we are no different from whatsoever it is that we eat in respect of the Loving Oneness shared with each and every organism and that in fact each and every seed contains the potential of awakening us to the Loving Oneness. It is a 'healthy' seed that will keep us healthy. In times of the Vedas, poisonous foods or else genetically altered foods did not exist nor did large scale produce of foods wrapped in plastics and tetra-packaging. Neither were animals slaughtered gruesomely, parts of which lie these days in supermarkets and our children at times do not even recognise which animal the meat is derived from. Illnesses like - among many others - cancer also did not exist in ancient times. Ayurveda reminds us to eat with grace. It means that we pay reverence to Mother Earth for offering us all foods, to the Sun and the Rains for their life-giving energies, to the farmers who harvest crops, and in fact to all those who help in bringing foods to our lives. Graciousness can be shown in many ways. We can help prepare meals, and assist in cleaning up after meals and it does not necessarily mean to pay reverence in connection to a religious doctrine.

Traditionally, a small portion of each food cooked was offered to the fire with reverence to *brahman*, considered to be the Lord and giver of all foods. The ancients of course did not know of microwave cooking, powdered foods, tetra-packaging, preservatives and food-colourings to satisfy the hunger of current times at its pace. We are, however, cautioned by the scientists and rishis of modern times in a way to take heed of many modern utensils or else forms of foods that are devoid of life-giving energy. Many of modern day electrical appliances aggravate the *vata dosha* and cause harm to the balance of '*tanmantra*' which is the energy quanta of food. Progressive transitions can gradually be made towards holistic healing. Some suggestions are to discard all frozen foods, canned foods, powdered foods and old spices as well as to become much more aware of maintaining variety in one's menu. These days there is also a vast variety of (affordable) organic foods.

Ayurveda suggests not to overeat but to eat the quantity that feels satisfying. The stomach may ideally be filled with 1/3 amount food, 1/3 liquids and kept 1/3 empty. Taking a small amount of warm water within half hour before a meal is also an Ayurvedic prescription to ignite one's digestive fire but drinking too much water during meals would have a contradictory effect. Regularity in meal timings is also recommended by the ancient rishis. Finally, one of the most important transitions one can make is to prepare food in peace and harmony and to consume food with a tranquil and silent mind.

> *"Earth, water, fire, air, space, manas (mind), buddhi (intellect), and ahamkara (ego) - these are the eight-fold divisions of my manifestation."*
> *Lord Krishna*

In Ayurveda, we can identify ourselves as a composition of the great five elements: ether, air, fire, water, and earth in our universe. Ether and air further combine into the doshas (humours), *Vata* (Ether + Air), *Pitta* (Fire) and *Kapha* (Water +Earth). Each of us and in fact each species on earth has all these five elements but in different quantities of *doshas.* It is best to consider how what we eat has an effect on the doshic equilibrium within ourselves. A lot of red chillies for instance, will increase the *pitta* or fire *dosha.* Once this correlation is recognised there can be no separation between us and our environment. These in themselves are the majestic forces of life which unless we remain in awareness and harmony will potentially bring about ill-health. Any excess or deficit of the humours leads to disease. Hence, it is important to consider what we eat and drink as well as how it is prepared.

Below is a list of foods and drinks suitable for all *dosha* (*Tridosha*) constitutional types:

VEGETABLES	Artichoke Asparagus Broccoli Carrots Corn, fresh Green beans	Mustard greens Onion, cooked Okra Parsley potatoes ,white Spinach	Sprouts Zucchini Sweet Potatoes Watercress
FRUITS	Apricots Berries Cherries Grapes, dark	Lemons Limes Mango Peaches	Pomegranate Raisins Strawberries, sweet Tamarind
NUTS & SEEDS	Nuts may be sparingly used	Pumpkin seeds	Sunflower seeds

GRAINS	Barley Basmati rice (brown & white) Millet Quinoa Wheat Oats, whole cooked Wild rice

PROCESSED GRAINS	Barley cereal & flour Bulguor Corn grits Cornmeal Couscous	Oats bran Pasta, spinach or whole wheat Rice flour	Wheat bran Whole wheat flour

	Millet cereal Mochi (pounded sweet rice)	Rye flakes and flour Soba noodles Udan noodles	

LEGUMES, BEANS, PEAS & SOYABEAN DERIVATIVES	Aduki beans Mung dhal, whole Tofu Urad dhal
SWEETENERS	Amasake (rice milk) Barley malt syrup Fruit juice concentrate Honey, raw and uncooked Maple syrup

HERBS, SPICES & FLAVOURINGS	Black pepper Cardamom Cinnamon Coconut Coriander Cilantro Cumin Dill leaves or seeds Fennel	Garlic, cooked Ghee Ginger, cooked Ginger, fresh Lemon Mint leaves Mustard Nutmeg Orange peel	Parsley Rose water Saffron Sea salt Tamarind Tarragon Turmeric Vanilla Wintergreen

DAIRY	Butter, unsalted Ghee Yoghurt, spiced Cottage cheese

OILS	Canola Sunflower

BEVERAGES	Aloe Vera juice Apple juice Apricot juice Amasake (rice milk)	Berry juices, sweet Carob drinks Carrot-vegetable juice Grape juice	Mango juice Peach nectar Soy milk, spiced Yoghurt drinks, spiced

TEAS	Barley (grain tea) Chamomile Chicory Cinnamon Cloves Elder flower Fennel	Hops Jasmine Lemon balm Lemon grass Lotus Mexican bark Orange peel	Peppermint Raspberry Rice (grain tea) Rose flower Saffron Spearmint Violet

The transition to healthy eating can easily be made gingerly and with a playful awareness of the five humours. The concept of humourism has unfortunately become far too discredited in modern times and medical sciences. It was however, abundant in ancient and medieval medicines and remained so for many centuries. The four humours were identified as black bile, yellow bile, phlegm, and blood. The Greeks and Romans, and the later Muslim and Western European medical establishments that adopted and adapted classical medical philosophy, also believed that each of these humours would wax and wane in the body, depending on diet and activity. Time and time again, centuries long, it has been respected that it is nature itself that contains healing powers, commonly known as "vis medicatrix naturae" or natura medica from the times of Hippocrates, the Greek 'father' of medicine. Since the time of the Vedas it has been understood that disease is dis-equilibrium of an organism and its environment and the prevention of disease would entail sustenance of a healthy equilibrium. Shamans too or other traditional healing systems like the hula medicine of the Hawaiian people recognise the natural and spiritual healing power of nature.

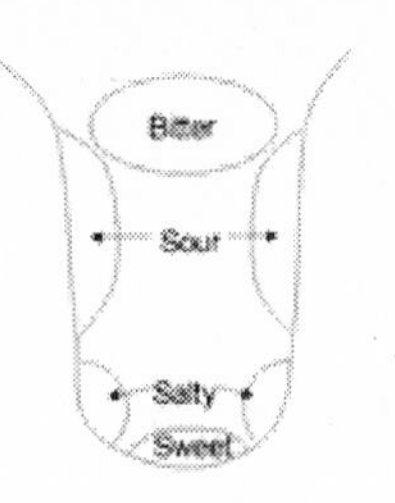

j jFigurejjRasasjonjTongue

The holistic principles of Ayurveda also know how to appreciate tastes in nature. The Sanskrit name for taste in Ayurveda is "Rasa" but *rasa* can also have a broader meaning. The term *rasa* refers to the complex chain of reactions that occur when we first register a perception made by one of our sense organs. This also includes how our brain cells in turn excite the appetite. Appetite is not just hunger but an overall intelligence of how our body acts in harmony with our environment. While food is desired, ingested, digested and ejected as waste, *rasa* is present in all the stages of this vital process. In the ordinary sense of its meaning, the six *rasas* or tastes include sweet, sour, pungent, salty, bitter and astringent.

As food enters our body, it signals an instantaneous heating or cooling response. This is called "virya" in Sanskrit. All pungent, sour and salty foods lead to a 'heating' virya. The amount of heat produced from the pungent taste is highest. Bitter, astringent and sweet foods yield to 'cooling' *virya*, and that produced by the bitter taste is lowest. Food is known in Ayurveda as "ausadam", translating as "that which is medicine". The rishis were able to define the properties and effects of food on us and the cause of disease. They made us aware that when food ceases to be medicine, medicine becomes impotent.

The post-digestive effect of food is called "vipaka", which is the ripening effect of its flavour. *Vipaka* is reduced in to three residual tastes sweet, sour and pungent from the six original tastes. Sweet remains sweet in its *vipaka* state, salty becomes sweet, sour remains sour and pungent, bitter, astringent leave a pungent *vipaka*. Below are charts that reflect and help clarify the doshas and their universal tastes as well as the beneficial tastes per *dosha*.

	DOSHAS & THEIR NATURAL TASTES	BENEFICIAL TASTES FOR EACH DOSHA
VATA	Bitter, astringent, pungent	Salty, sour, sweet
PITTA	Sour, salty, pungent	Bitter, astringent, sweet
KAPHA	Sweet, sour, salty	Pungent, bitter, astringent

In the *doshas*, *vata*, *pitta*, *kapha*, the principle of like increases like applies which means that the inherent taste of each dosha will be reinforced if that *dosha* is fed its own tastes. This does not mean that each *dosha* type should only eat foods and tastes that are best for its own body type. In fact all three *doshas* are present and benefit everyone and hence a combination of all six tastes is necessary in a person's diet. Recognising the effects of rasa on *doshas*, however, is the key to harmonising the *doshas*, keeping them in balance and (*vipaka*) which reduces into the three residual tastes sweet, sour and pungent and results in "ojas". *Ojas* is thus, the nutritive plasma that feeds the organs and tissues of the body after digestion and after assimilation is completed. When appropriate lifestyle, seasonal influences, healthy food and mental calm is not maintained, *ojas* is diminished. This weakens the body's auto-immune system making it vulnerable to disease.

Ayurveda also enjoins us to take heed of incompatible foods. These are:

Dairy products and salts or salted foods.

Dairy products and animal foods (especially fish).

Fruits and any other foods.

Hot and cold foods.

Hot oil and butter.

Ghee and honey in equal quantity.

Heated honey and ingestion of alkaline food for long periods is also not recommended. Ideally, it is best to maintain a balance of alkaline and acid from foods. Generally, most meat, fish, white sugar, peanuts, white pasta and alcohol have an extremely high acid content while garlic, ginger, curry powder, cinnamon, broccoli, carrot, alfalfa, sunflower seeds, nettle tea, apples, grapefruits, melons have an extremely high alkaline content.

Following is an overview of *rasa* and its effects:

RASA (Initial taste)	*VIPAKA* (Post-digestive taste)	EFFECT	MAIN FUNCTION
Sweet	Sweet	Increases K decreases V, P	Increases body tissues
Sour	Sour	Increases K, P decreases V	Increases appetite
Salty	Sweet	Increases K, P decreases V	Makes body limber and cleanses the body
Pungent	Pungent	Increases P, V decreases K	Reduces fluid in tissues
Bitter	Pungent	Increases V decreases P, K	Purifies organs and controls skin ailments
Astringent	Pungent	Increases V Decreases P, K	Purifies and constricts body

Finally, Charaka has advised us on ten factors to consider on the subject of diet for our well-being:

1) One should take warm food as this not only makes the food delicious but also aids in overall digestion.
2) One should take unctuous food as it also makes food delicious but also provokes subdued power of digestion.
3) One should take a balanced quantity of food to promote longevity.
4) One should take a meal only when the previous meal is properly digested otherwise the balance of our humours goes astray.
5) One should take food having no contradictory potencies, like hot and cold.

6) One should take food in a proper environment.
7) One should not eat and swallow food too fast.
8) One should also not take food too slowly as this may feel unsatisfactory.
9) One should eat with concentration rather than to be excessively talking or laughing.
10) One should regard the food one is eating and recognise its essence for our self-preservation.

Chapter Seven

Ethical Care

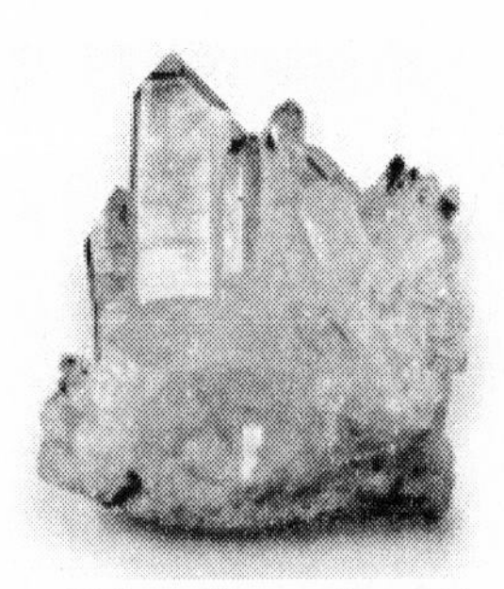

j jFigurejjQuartzjCrystal

Charaka-Samhita tells us that mind, objects of mind, intellect and soul are all substances and qualities pertaining to the Self. This entire group is inclined towards or else abstaining from auspicious and inauspicious acts and that whatever actions we take can be therapeutic in nature or upsetting. We perceive everything through the predominance of *akasa*, *vayu*, *tejas*, *ap*, *prthivi* (the five elements) and there is derangement when these are not in a balanced or a normalcy level. This becomes the basis for Ayurveda's ethical care.

The sages of Ayurveda have shared that whilst mind seems to be more than one because of the variations in its own objects, sense objects, its analytical activity and also its conjunction with *rajas*, *tamas* and *sattva*, in fact, (one) mind does not attend to more than one thing at a time. The sages also tell us that our sense organs are only capable of perceiving their objects when they are supported by mind and that it is important to consider the qualities which are predominant and time and again present in the mind. So, in order to prevent derangements in the mind along with sense organs, it is recommended to make effort to maintain normalcy by means of embracing wholesome acts and thoughts and (re)examining with intellect, self-reflection towards good conduct.

The ancient texts of Charaka Samhita suggests that "One should worship gods, cow, *Brahmanas*, preceptors, elderly people, accomplished and teachers. One should honour fire, one should put auspicious herbs, one should wash twice a day, one should clean excretory passages and feet frequently; cutting hair, shaving and nail cutting should be done thrice a fortnight; one should always wear untorn clothes, use flowers and fragrance; dress should be gentle and style of hair as commonly practised, one should apply oil on head, ear, nose and feet daily; should not smoke, should take initiative in talk and remain cheerful, one should have presence of mind even in difficult circumstances, perform religious sacrifices, donate, pay respect to road crossings, offer religious offerings, entertain guests, offer rice balls to forefathers, one should speak useful, measured, sweet and meaningful words; should be self-controlled, self-virtuous, jealous in cause and not in effect, free from anxiety, fearless, shy, wise, great and courageous, skilful, forbearing, religious, positivist, devoted to teachers, accomplished persons and who are superior in modesty, intellect, learning, clan and age. One should walk having umbrella, stick, turban and footwear and looking six feet forward. One should adopt auspicious conduct, should avoid places with dirty cloth, bones, thorns, impure articles, hairs, chaff, garbage, ash, skull, and of bath and sacrifice. One should discontinue exercise before fatigue, one should behave like kith and kin to all living beings, pacify the angry, console the frightened, help the poor, be truthful, peaceful, tolerant of other's harsh words, remover of intolerance, should always look at the qualities of peaceful life and should alleviate the causes of attachment and aversion. One should not tell a lie nor should take over other's possession nor should desire for other women or other's property."

Naturally, while many of the guidelines laid out by our ancients remain of considerable value in modern times, some such as "offering rice balls to our forefathers" might seem farfetched to some these days. These, nonetheless, need not undermine the overall direction given to us for virtuous conduct which if nothing else offers grandeur, loving and harmonious psychological well-being - in other words, "true to the heart".

One of the most valuable of all practices is that of Ahimsa. This appears in the Yajur Veda and later in one of the oldest and primary Upanishads called the "Chanddogya Upanishads" dated to the 8th and 17th century BC. *Ahimsa* means the avoidance of violence. The Sanskrit term *Ahimsa* means 'to do no harm'. It believes that all forms of violence against all creatures create negative consequences or *karma*. Following the path of *Ahimṣa* encourages one to improve ourselves rather than the focus being on improving the world and to take a vow for *Ahimsa* so as to end the battle within one's own mind that ends up in conflict, hatred, ambition, anger and more such negative states. Following *Ahimsa* can help to make life transforming choices. You can ask yourself the question: Does this decision or choice support inner Harmony?" The answers to this question can become the steps towards Divine Love and harmony, which is the very essence of the Vedas. In *Ahimsa* meditation you learn to become 'watchful' of any negative or bothersome thought rather than 'to act' upon it. In this way you merely become a witness and offer it to the cosmic space of *Ahimsa.* This way you learn objectivity and to see situations for what they really are. Finally, a solution becomes clear with awareness. *Ahimsa* can also to be practiced in speech.

Words cannot describe the joy of the spirit whose spirit is cleansed in deep contemplation--who is one with his/her own Spirit (of Ahimsa). Only those who experience this joy know what it is.

--Maitri Upanishad

Words can lead us to hate or love, conflict or to peace. Hitler used words to lead millions unto death and destruction while Jesus used his for love and compassion. The Vedic scriptures caution us that we can take our voices for granted and tend to use it for abuse in the most trivial of our mundane lives. The Vedic scriptures tell us that if there are no words there would in fact be no knowledge of right and wrong, pleasing and unpleasing. The words in fact make this all known. The voice is in fact an extension of our prana, life giving energy, and meant to love and not to hurt. Should a negative thought arise, it is best to write it down and finally redirect it unto ourselves. Ahimsa helps us realize that hurting another is in fact hurting ourselves.

Practicing *Ahimsa* is the main yamas or "restraints "out of the ten offered to us by the rishis as a path to live virtuously, lovingly, harmoniously and joyfully in resonance with our inherit natural selves. *Yama* is Sanskrit for the lord of death, whose first recorded appearance is in the Vedas. He is also one of the most ancient beings in the world and parallel forms of one sort or another are found all over Eurasia. He is also known as Yima by Zoroastrians, and is considered to be cognate with Ymir of Norse legend and has become known as Enma, or Emma-o, in Japanese legend. *Yama* represents the lord of *Yama* justice and is sometimes referred to as *Dharma*, in reference to his unswerving dedication to maintaining order and adherence to harmony.

The ten *yama*-restraints are:

1) *Ahimsa* - abstinence from injury, harmlessness, not causing of pain to any living creature in thought, word, or deed at any time.
2) *Satya* - Truthfulness in living and speaking words of truth and non-coveting, non-stealing,
3) *Aparigraha* - To lose one's peace of mind in chasing after or bounding oneself to material wealth and fame), practicing

4) *Brahmacharya* - divine conduct, faithful when married) are regarded as Yama or constraints
5) *Kshama:* patience, releasing time, functioning in the now.
6) *Dhriti:* steadfastness, overcoming non-perseverance, fear, and indecision; seeing each task through to completion.
7) *Daya:* compassion; conquering callous, cruel and insensitive feelings toward all beings.
8) *Arjava:* honesty, straightforwardness, renouncing deception and wrongdoing.
9) *Mitahara:* moderate appetite, neither eating too much nor too little; nor consuming meat, fish, shellfish, fowl or eggs.
10) *Shaucha:* purity, avoidance of impurity in body, mind and speech.

These are also versed in the Yoga sutras of Patanjali. As Ayurveda precedes all spiritual guidelines in time, we must recognize that almost all of the *yamas* have been rephrased and brought to us afresh by many enlightened persons up-to-date.

The ancients' texts also advise us to practice niyama, which are more religious in practice. The ten *niyamas* are:

1) *Hri*: "Remorse." Being modest and showing shame for misdeeds.
2) *Santosha*: "Contentment." Seeking joy and serenity in life.
3) *Dana*: "Giving." Tithing and giving generously without thought of reward.
4) *Astikya*: (Sanskrit) "Faith." Believing firmly in God, Gods, guru and the path to enlightenment.
5) *Ishvarapujana*: "Worship of the Lord." The cultivation of devotion through daily worship and meditation.
6) *Siddhanta shravana*: "Scriptural listening." Studying the teachings and listening to the wise of one's lineage.

7) *Mati*: "Cognition." Developing a spiritual will and intellect with the guru's guidance.
8) *Vrata*: "Sacred vows." Fulfilling religious vows, rules and observances faithfully.
9) *Japa*: "Recitation." Chanting mantras daily.
10) *Tapas*: "Austerity." Performing *sadhana*, penance, *tapas* and sacrifice.

Patanjali lists the *yamas* as non covetousness and the *niyamas* as self-reflection, scriptural study and worship. Ayurveda guides us to embrace as many codes or virtuous conduct along with the guidelines of daily and seasonal routine so that we may live joyously and in a healthy way with our environment. One of the most beautiful of all advises from the rishis is to embrace the essence of loving silence, it being our true nature. Unnecessarily wasting our breath in a way depletes us from our vital energies. The greatest sadhana or spiritual practice is to sit in the true nature of our own being, in love, light and watchfulness. All that is needed for this is a few moments of our time.

Conclusion

Ayurveda is sacred timeless loving wisdom. It lays the platform of taking charge of our well-being and nourishes our awareness of the Divine. It is holistic in its nurturing our body, mind and soul. It asks us to live in harmony with ourselves and our environment as part of the same universe. It brings us closer to our true nature of peace and loving harmony. Rather than to focus on disease, Ayurveda brings us back to our inherent state of good health and equilibrium.

The longing for our well-being and to live in harmony with our environment has been practised for centuries by many a people unto our present times. The peoples of yesterday were breathing the same air as today, were bathing in the same sunlight as today and were waiting for the rainfall to shower upon crops just like today. However, many of us have forgotten how to live in harmony within ourselves and our environment. While the ancient rishis brought forth the universal wisdom of Ayurveda more than 5000 years ago, the rishis of today can and do exist in support of holistic wisdom. We only need to awaken our cosmic memory and rekindle divine wisdom within ourselves. We can in fact prevent this from happening before we or our planet becomes unwell.

This book has marked the importance of Ayurvedic daily, seasonal and ethical routines to help us preserve our inner balance. It has in fact become crucial in modern times of terrorism and pollution. We need to closely consider the choices we make in our lives and we need not look anywhere else but within ourselves. We need not eat foods that are filled with toxins. We need not exhaust our senses in fear of what we find on the media. We need not wake up one day wondering why we are so unwell.

Ayurveda has brought us the wisdom that everything in life has five elements in different proportions; ether, air, fire, water and earth. Each of these elements has their own qualities. We also have the three energies of *sattva*, *rajas* and *tamas*. We are also made up of *Buddhi* or ego and of *Atma*, or soul. In following the daily, seasonal and ethical routines we can maintain our health and well-being in a physical, mental but also spiritual perspective. This is essential in Ayurveda not only after we have undergone treatment but for prevention of illness. Following the daily, seasonal and ethical routines are fundamental to living a life of harmony and balance and joy.

Recipes of Sattvic Foods

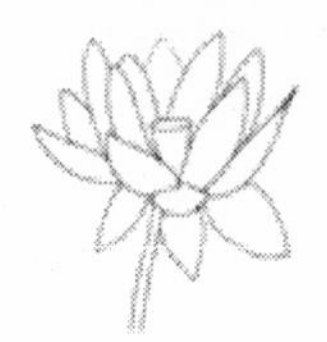

Ghee (ghrta, sarpi) – Good for all *doshas*

1 bar of unsalted organic butter
A stainless steel frying pan

Melt and allow the butter to cook in the frying pan gently over a moderate flame for about 10-15 minutes. Watch carefully to avoid burning while allowing the foam to surface during the heating process to settle in to sediment. When the ghee begins to boil silently, with only a trace of air bubbles then the ghee is ready. Allow the ghee to cool and pour in to a clean container for storage leaving behind the sediment in the frying pan.

Ghee is known to be one of the most *Sattvic* foods in Ayurveda. It is ideal for cooking as it does not burn unless of course excessively heated.

"It promotes memory, intelligence, agni - vital fire, semen, ojas – vital essence, kapha and fat. It is curative of Vata, Pitta, fever and toxins". Charaka

Khichadi - Good for all *doshas*

Khichadi is a mixture of grains and beans which is easy to digest and nourishing. It is often given during Ayurvedic cleansing therapies.

Servings for two:

1 cup white or brown basmati rice

½ cup whole mung dhal

8 cups of boiling water (and less if a thicker khichadi is desired)

1 tbs ghee

1 tsp black pepper corns

1tsp ground cumin seeds

½ tsp ginger (even less for pitta constitution types)

Pinch of salt

Pinch of turmeric powder

Soak mung beans in water for a couple of hours. Add ghee in to a large pan and sauté the peppercorns, cumin seeds and ginger for some moments. Add rice and beans in to the mixture and sauté again for 2-3 minutes. Add boiling water, turmeric and salt. Cover and simmer gently for an hour on low heat stirring occasionally.

Warm Almond Saffron Milk – Good for all *doshas* and best taken in the evening or before bedtime

Servings for two:

1 cup milk

1 ½ cup water

Six almonds

Few strands of saffron

Soak the almonds over night. Combine milk and water and bring to boil. Add crushed almonds and saffron and simmer for a few minutes.

Lettuce Salad with Fresh Mint– Good for all *doshas*

Servings for two

About 12 lettuce leaves

6 leaves of mint

½ tsp salt

½ tsp sesame seeds

A pinch of ginger powder

2 tbs sesame oil

Sesame seeds

Sesame oil

Toss lettuce with salt and leave aside for one hour. Add sesame seeds and ginger to the sesame oil to make a dressing. Pour the dressing over the lettuce and finally add chopped mint.

Lassi with Rosewater and Walnuts – Good for all *doshas*

Servings for two

1 ½ cups of water

1 ½ cups of milk

¼ cup yoghurt

¼ cup ground walnuts

2 tbs honey

1 tbs rosewater

Place all ingredients in a blender and blend for a few minutes until smooth.

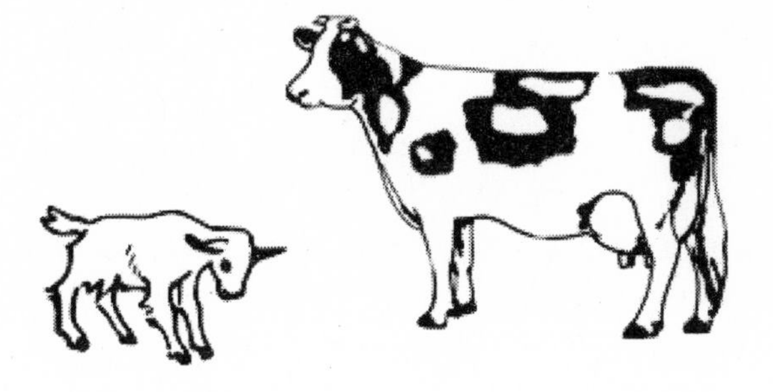

Missi Roti with Spinach – Good for all *doshas*

Servings for two

1 cup whole wheat flour

1 cup corn flour

1 tbs ghee

¾ cup water

¼ cup spinach

¼ tsp salt

Combine flour and salt and ghee and mix with finger tips. Add half water and boiled spinach and knead the dough for about 5 minutes. Add the remaining water and knead for another 5 minutes. Cover with a damp cloth and allow resting for 2 hours. Divide dough in to 12 small pieces.

Lightly flour a clean surface of a table and use your hands to press each dough pieces in to patties. Roll out each patty on the floured surface to enlarge, adding some extra flour as required to the surface.

Preheat a griddle and cook roti on each side for about 30 seconds on medium heat. Remove gentle with tongs.

Yogi Tea – Good for all *doshas*

Servings for 2

1 small thumb of crushed ginger

2 small cinnamon sticks

6 small cardamom pods

½ tsp fennel seeds

6 cloves

1 half tsp black tea

1¼ cup water

1 cup milk

2 tsp honey

Break the cinnamon sticks in to small pieces and cook in boiling water with all the other spices and tea for 2-3 minutes. Add milk and allow cooking for another 1-2 minutes. Serve with honey.

Digestive Aid Spice Mix – Good for all *doshas*

Qty. 6 ounces

2 oz. whole fennel seeds

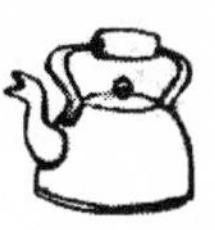

2 oz. whole cumin seeds or powder

2 oz. ground coriander seeds

Add ingredients in to a 8 oz. glass jar, close lid and mix well. This spice mix can be used as spices in meals or consumed as tea. In the case of tea, the spices should be ground and one tablespoon can be added to one cup of hot water.

Properties of Gems

NB Gems can be purified by placing them in water with a pinch of salt overnight as well as by occasionally exposing them to direct sunlight.

Amethyst – Purple or blue. Amethyst offers love, compassion and hope. It is good for healing and for balancing out one's emotions. It also gives individual dignity. It is a very good help against addictions. It realigns and readjusts disorders. It can best be worn around the neck on a gold necklace. It mainly contains the elements ether and water and is best for *vata* and *pitta* imbalances.

Diamond – White, blue or red. Diamonds are good for the heart and brain. It is considered to be a heart tonic. This tonic can be made by placing a diamond in a glass of water overnight and drinking it the next day. Diamonds rallies strength with age.

Diamonds bring prosperity and a feeling of spiritual uplifting. It brings people closer to one another. It can best be worn on the right ring finger in a gold ring. Diamonds mainly contain the elements ether, air, fire, water and earth. Red diamond stimulates *pitta.* Blue diamond calms pitta and stimulates *kapha.* Colourless diamond stimulates *vata* and *kapha* and calms *pitta.*

NB Diamonds of low quality can have a negative effect on the body.

Garnet – Red, brown, black, green, yellow and white. Red, brown and yellow garnets are beneficial for *vata* and *kapha* disorders. White and green are useful for *pitta* disorders. Garnet can best be worn around the neck in a gold setting for *vata* and *kapha*. For *pitta*, a silver setting is preferable.

Red garnet mainly has fire and earth elements; green garnet mainly has fire and air elements and white garnet mainly has the water element.

Lapis Lazuli – Blue, violet or green. Lapis Lazuli strengthens the eyes and is beneficial for various eye diseases. It also gives strength to the body and mind and helps to increase sensitivity to higher spiritual vibrations. It is a heavenly, sacred stone. It can best be worn around the neck on a gold necklace. Lapis Lazuli mainly contains the elements ether, fire and water. It is good for *vata* and *kapha*.

Pearl – White, black. Pearl has strengthening qualities and promotes vitality. Pearl is also a very good blood purifier. In its ash form, it can be used internally for stomach and intestinal inflammatory diseases. It may also be employed in the treatment of hepatitis and gall stones. Pearl also has haemostatic properties and can therefore be used in the treatment of bleeding gums, vomiting with bleeding or bleeding piles.

The electrical energy of pearl water may be harnessed by making pearl water. Pearl water can be made by placing four or five pearls in a glass of water and kept overnight. This water can be taken as a tonic the next day and can help in alleviating burning sensation in the eyes as well as urine.

Pearl can best be worn on the right ring finger in a silver ring. Pearl mainly contains water, air and earth and has anti-*pitta* properties.

Red coral is red and is known to absorb energy from the planet Mars. It is a blood purifier and it helps to calm anger, hate and jealousy. It is best worn around the neck in a gold chain or else in a gold ring on the right index finger.

Red coral mainly has the elements water, earth and fire and generally calms *pitta.*

Ruby – Red, pink. Ruby strengthens the heart. It also helps in concentration and mental power. It can be worn either in gold or a silver ring on the left ring finger. Ruby mainly contains the elements fire, air and ether and calms *pitta.*

Sapphire – Violet, purple or black. Violet helps in diseases like sciatica, rheumatism, neurological pain, epilepsy, hysteria and generally most *vata* ailments. It is used to counter act the negative effects of the planet Saturn. It can best be worn in a gold setting around the neck. It mainly contains the elements air and ether.

Quartz Crystal – are in numerous forms. They are generally very good metaphysical aids in amplifying positive energy and transmuting negative energy. Crystals help balance the flow of subtle energies in the physical and subtle bodies.

Tourmaline – are in numerous forms. Black tourmaline is particularly good in amplifying positive energy and transmuting negative energies. It repels radiation expelled from computer monitors and other appliances. It is connected to the base *chakra,* helps in increasing "grounding" and was commonly used both by the Native American Indians as well as by African Shamans to help awaken from "dreams of illusions". Black tourmaline also helps against anxiety, heart disease, arthritis and dyslexia.

Properties of Metals

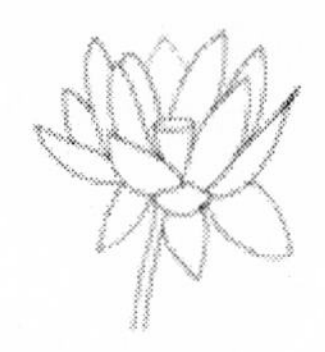

NB Metals potentially have toxic effects when used in excess and must never be used without supervision of a qualified Ayurvedic physician.

Gold is an effective nervine tonic. It improves memory, intelligence, increases stamina and strengthens the muscles of the heart. Gold (water) is beneficial for treating hysteria epilepsy, heart attacks and a weak liver and spleen.

The energy of gold can be harnessed through the use of medicated gold water. This can be made by placing a gold ornament (without any stone) into two glasses of water and then boiling it until half the water evaporates. One teaspoon of this water may be taken twice or thrice a day.

Gold has heating properties and must be used with caution for *pitta* constitutions.

Silver has cooling properties and is beneficial for treating excess *pitta*. It is also used for *vata* ailments. Silver promotes strength and stamina and works well against chronic fever, weakness after fever and heartburn. It also helps in inflammatory conditions of the intestines, profuse menstrual bleeding and hyperactivity of the gall bladder. Silver water can be prepared in the same manner as gold water. Drinking warm milk heated in a silver container improves strength and stamina. Silver is best used for *pitta* and *vata* constitutions.

Copper is good for *kapha* constitutions. It alleviates excess fat and is a good tonic for the heart, spleen and lymphatic system. It helps in curing anaemia as well. Copper is beneficial for a person who tends to put on weight, retains water or has a lymphatic obstruction. Copper (water) helps against obesity, liver or spleen disorders. It is best to wear a copper bracelet on the wrist. Copper water can be made by placing some copper pennies or bracelet in to lime water and in one quarter water. This should then be boiled until half the water evaporates. Two teaspoons of this water should be taken thrice a day for one month.

Iron is beneficial for red bloods cells, liver, spleen, bone marrow and bone tissue. It increases the levels of red blood cells. It also helps strengthen muscle and nerve tissues and has rejuvenating properties. Iron ash is effectively used to treat anaemia and enlargement of the liver or spleen.

Properties of Colours

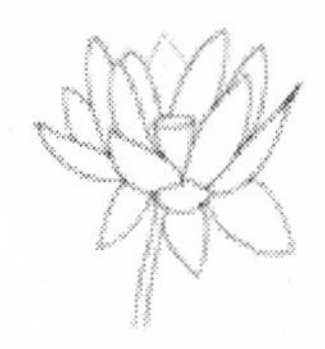

NB The seven colours of the rainbow are beneficial for all three constitutions. A gelatinous paper of any of the seven colours of the rainbow can be wrapped around a jar of water and placed in the sunlight for four hours. The water will then become infused by the vibrations of that colour.

Red is related to blood. It promotes the colour of red in red blood cells and stimulates the formation of red blood cells. It also gives lustre to the skin as well as energy to the nerve tissue and bone marrow. Red has heating properties and calms excess *vata* and *kapha*. On the other hand, overexposure to red can cause *pitta* in the body to increase. Overuse can cause conjunctivitis.

Yellow stimulates understanding and intelligence. In terms of spiritual terms, yellow causes death of the ego. It is connected with the crown *chakra*. Yellow calms *vata* and kapha and has heating properties. Excess of yellow can cause excess of bile to collect in the small intestine.

Green is connected to the heart *chakra*. It calms the mind and soothes emotions bringing happiness within the heart. It calms *vata* and *kapha* and aggravates *pitta*. Excess of green can cause abundance of bile which in turn may create stones to collect in the gall bladder.

Blue has a peaceful and soothing effect on the mind and the body. It is connected with Pure Consciousness. It relieves liver diseases and aggravates *pitta.* At the same time, excess use of blue can aggravate *vata* and *kapha.*

Violet lightens the body and deepens our sense of perception. It is connected to Cosmic Consciousness. It calms excess *pitta* and *kapha* but can aggravate *vata.*

Prakrti

Ayurvedic Dosha/Constitution test

By filling out the following tables you can derive your Ayurvedic Constitution, known as *Prakrti.* Select the answer that you feel suits you best from the column *vata*, *pitta* or *kapha.* Add a V-P-K respectfully in the column. The sum total of either V, P or K will give you your *Prakrti.* The highest sum total is your main *dosha.* In case the sum total of another *dosha* is also high, then it means that your *Prakrti* is a combination of two *doshas* with one being more dominant.

OBSERVATIONS	*VATA*	**V**	*PITTA*	**P**	*KAPHA*	
Body size	Thin build		Medium build		Large build	
Body weight	Low		Medium		Heavy side	
Weight change	Trouble gaining		Can gain but lose quickly		Gains weight easily, hard to lose	
Skin type	Thin, dry		Smooth, combination skin		Thick, oily,	
Skin texture	Cold, roughness, light colour		Warm, reddish, freckles		Cool, pale	
Hair	Dry, brittle, scarce, gets knotted		Straight, oily, prone to hair loss		Thick, curly, oily, wavy, luxuriant	
Hair colour	Brown, black		Blond, gray, red,		Dark black, dark brown	
Nose	Uneven shape, deviated septum		Long, pointed, red nose tip		Short, rounded, button nose	
Eyes	Small, sunken, dry, active, and possibly freq. blinking		Sharp, sensitive to light		Big, calm,	
Eye colour	Black, brown		Gray, green, yellow, red		Blue, light	
Nails	Dry, rough, easily broken		Sharp, flexible, long, reddish tint		Thick, smooth, shiny surface	
Lip	Dry, cracked		Often inflamed		Smooth, large	

Lip colour	Black or brown tint		Red or yellowish		Pale	
Chin	Thin and angular		Tapered		Rounded, big	
Cheeks	Sunken, lines or wrinkles		Flat and smooth		Big or round	
Neck	Long, thin		Medium		Wide	
Chest	Small, flat		Moderate		Broad chested	
Belly	Small, flat		Moderate		large, defined	
Hips	Small or thin		Moderate		Big	
Joints	Cracking noise		Moderate		Large, lubricated	
Appetite	Irregular in frequency and magnitude		Strong, cannot skip meals		Steady, regular	
Taste preference	Sweet, sour, salty		Sweet, bitter, astringent		Bitter, pungent, astringent	
Thirst	Variable		Need water regularly		Sparse need for water	
Digestion	Irregular		Quick		Slow	
When there is indigestion	Tendency to constipation, forms gas		Causes burning, heart burn, reflux		Forms mucous	
Elimination	Dry		Loose		Thick, sluggish	
Physical activity	Always active		Moderate		Slow, measured	
Mental activity	Always active		Moderate		Calm	

Personality	Vivacious, talkative, social, outgoing		Likes to be in control, purpose based interaction		Reserved, laid back, concerned	
Emotional response when stressed	Anxiety, fear		Anger, hate, jealousy		Greedy, possessive, withdrawn	
Faith or beliefs	Variable		Dedicated/extreme		Consistent	
Intellectual response	Quick, not detailed		Accurate, timely		Paced but exact	
Memory	Good short term, quick to forget		Medium but accurate		Slow to remember but then sustained	
Career, life preference	Creative arts, designing		Science or engineering		Management, human relations, care giving	
Environment	Easily feels cold		Intolerant of heat		Uncomfortable in humidity	
Sleep	Short, broken up		moderate and sound		Deep and long	
Dreams	Multiple and quick, fearful		Fiery, often about conflicts		Slow, romantic	
Speech	Rapid, hither thither		precise, articulate		Slow, monotonous	
Financial	Buy on impulse		Spends money on luxuries		Good at saving money	
Total VPK						

Glossary

Agni – Digestive fire and one of the five main cosmic elements

Ahimsa – Non-violence, non-harming, abstinence from harmful thought, speech and action

Ama – Toxins in the digestive tract as a result of bad digestion

Ap – Sanskrit for water, as one of the five main cosmic elements/humours

Atharva Veda – Atharvan's knowledge; one of the four Vedic hymn collections that is mainly about magical spells, rituals and yoga

Ausadam – Means that which is medicine

Ayurveda – Science of Life, Wisdom of Life; a holistic system of medicine and recommendations for healthy living derived from the Atharva and the Rig-Veda, dating back up to 5000 years ago.

Bandha – Bandhas are a small but important group of yogic practices. The Sanskrit word *bandha* means 'to hold' or "to lock" which are the action necessary to perform these practices.

Brahman – Absolute Consciousness (Brahma is different from Brahman which means the Creator)

Charaka Samhita – Ayurvedic texts related to internal medicine. These are compiled by Charaka dating back roughly to the 3rd century BC. 'Charaka' means wandering physicians' and 'Samhita' means 'collected *sutras* or formula'.

Dhanvantari – The physician of Gods and of Ayurveda. He is regarded as the source of Ayurveda and known to be the earliest medical practitioner and surgeon. He is also a descendant of Lord Vishnu, the supreme soul, in Hinduism.

Dharma – from '*dhri*' which means 'to sustain, carry, or hold'. *Dharma* is the inherent nature of human beings and their fulfilment of (divine) destiny. It concerns living in accordance to the law of nature, virtue and truth.

Dincharya – Daily routine, guidelines

Dosha – literally means 'flaws or faults' and relates to one of the three forces that emerges from the five elements or humours within the body

Ganthis – Psychic blocks and mental problems which prevent a person from properly experiencing higher states of awareness. *Ganthis* can be effectively removed by yogic practices called *Bandhas*.

Gayatri Mantra – is celebrated as one the greatest of all the mantras. It is originally from the Rig Vedas. It is addressed to the Sun as a form of Divine Light. Gayatri is also the Mother of the Vedas and protects those who recite this *mantra*.

Ghrita – Ghee, clarified butter and considered to be the primary elixir of good health.

Gunas – Prime qualities of nature as *sattva*, *rajas* and *tamas*

Humours – Five basic substances or elements that make up the body based on humourism. It is believed that when these substances are in balance then the body is in balance. All excess or deficit of these humours results in disease. These elements, in Ayurveda, are ether, air, fire, water and earth. Later, Greek, Roman, Muslim and Western European forms of medicines also adopted humourism.

Hatha yoga – 'Yoga of force'; the yoga for mental, physical, emotional and spiritual well-being.

Kala – Time, period

Kapha – Biological water and earth element, humour.

Kappalabhati – Means 'skull lustre'; *Kapāla* means skull *Bhāti* means light. This exercise gets its name because when practising the mind fills with a bright light. A combination of three practices to clear passages of breath, to give beauty and vitality.

Lassi – Spiced yoghurt drink often used after meals to aid in digestion.

Mantra – Sacred and mystical sounds for meditation and healing. Reciting *mantras* enforces and energetic field of protection.

Manas – Mind

Milarepa – Jetsun Milarepa (c. 1052-1135 CE) is known for his songs and writings on Tibetan Mahayana Buddhism. He is Tibet's most well-known yogi and poet.

Mudra – Means 'seal'; a sacred hand gesture which denote specific powers of energy.

Ojas – Means 'glow of health'; essence of the human body's endurance and immunity.

Pancha Karma – means 'five actions'. Pancha Karma is believed by practitioners to have a rejuvenating effect. This five-fold therapy is aimed at Shodhana, the eradication of the basic cause of disease. Shodhana or eradication, along with Shamana, the mitigation of the disease and its symptoms, are the two main concepts of disease management in Ayurveda. The five therapies are Nasya (Nasal therapy), *Vamana* (Emesis), *Virechana* (Purgation), *Vasti* (Enema) and *Raktamokshana* (Blood letting for purification of blood).

Pantajali – is the compiler of the 'Yoga Sutras', an important collection on the practice of yoga. Pantajali lived around the turn of the 1st and 2nd century BC.

Pitta – Biological Fire element, humour.

Prana – From the root '*Pran*' which means 'to breathe'; primary or vital life force.

Pranayama – Extending of *prana*, breath control exercises.

Prithvi – Earth, as one of the five main cosmic elements.

Rajas – Guna, quality of movement, activity.

Rasa – Juice, plasma, lymph.

Rig Veda – The oldest and most sacred collection of Vedic hymns and means "knowledge of praise. Rishis – Seers; a term for an enlightened being or a wise, psychic or visionary person.

Rtucharya – Seasonal routine, guidelines.

Rtusandhi – Junctions between seasons when susceptibility to illness is high.

Sadhanas – Spiritual gestures, practices.

Sattva – Guna, quality of purity, harmony, balance and naturally peaceful.

Shatkarmas – Yogic cleansing practices.

Shruti – That which is heard; cosmic revelation of what is heard, seen and articulated by Vedic seers.

Sushruta Samhita – A compilation of Ayurvedic texts attributed to Sushruta, the historical sage physician dating back to 1599 BC. Sushruta is known to be the "father of surgery". The texts as preserved date back to the 3rd and 4th century AD. The chapters include descriptions of 1120 illnesses, 700 medicinal plants, a thorough study of anatomy, 64 mineral based preparations and 57 on animal sources.

Tamas – *Guna* or cosmic force, quality of inertia.

Tanmantra – the five subtle properties of Energy or Matter; ether, air, fire, water and earth.

Tejas – Main form of fire element, humour *Pitta*, also brilliant energy or pure consciousness within the body.

Tridosha – *vata*, *pitta* and *kapha*.

Upanishad – means 'sitting near'; they constitute the core teachings of yoga and form the first comprehensive texts on yoga. They do not belong to a specific period. The Sanskrit term upani is derive from *uda*-(nearby), *ni*- (at the proper place, down) and *sad*, that is "sitting down near" a teacher in order to receive instruction.

Vata – Biological ether and air element, humour.

Vayu – Form of *prana* or *vata* and principle form of kinetic energy.

Vedanta - Yoga was presented symbolically until it first took a more definable shape in the Upanishads and finally collectively formed the Vedanta.

Vedas – A compilation of a large selected of sacred texts from ancient India. They are written in Vedic Sanskrit. The texts are an aggregate of four canonical "Samhitas" or Vedas. The four main Vedas are the Rig Veda containing hymns recited by the chief priest, the Yajur Veda contains formulae to be recited by the officiating priest, the Sam Veda, contains formulae to be chanted by Vedic priests specialised in soma practice, i.e. essence of plants, the Atharva Veda is a collection of spells, stories, predictions and apotropaic charms.

Vipaka – is the post-digestive effect of food. It is the ripening effect of its flavour. *Vipaka* is reduced in to three residual tastes sweet, sour and pungent from the six original tastes.

Virya – *Virya* is the instantaneous heating or cooling response of food as it enters our body.

Yama – "Lord of Death' – *Yamas* are restraints that one performs while practising *Ahimsa*.

Yoga – from the root '*yuj*' which means 'to unite or to join'; a spiritual practice to merge body, mind and spirit with the inner and outer universe.

Bibliography

Books:

"Ayurveda; A Life of Balance" by Maya Tiwari, ISBN 0-89281-676-1 – Inner Traditions India 1995.

"Ayurveda; Secrets of Healing" by Maya Tiwari, ISBN 978-81208-1452-3 – Lotus Press 1995.

"Ayurveda; The Science of Self-Healing – A Practical Guide" by Dr Vasant Lad, ISBN 81-208-1130-5 – Motilal Banarsida Publishers Private Ltd. Delhi.

"Leven met de seizoenen" by Patricia F. Wessels, ISBN 8-711776-641077 – Weleda.

"A systematic course in the ancient tantric techniques of yoga and kriya" by Swami Satyananda Saraswati, Published by G. K. Kejriwal Bihar 1981.

"Hatha Yoga Pradipika" by Swami Muktibodhananda, ISBN 978-81-85787-38-1 – Bihar School of Yoga, 1998 3rd edition.

"Hatha Yoga" by Juliet Pegrum, ISBN 1-903116-78-3, Cico Books 2003.

"Light on yoga" by BKS Iyengar, ISBN 81-7223-501-1 – HarperCollins Publishers India, 31st publication 2005

"The Ayurveda Encyclopaedia" by Swami Sada Shiva Tirtha, ISBN 978-81-319-0309-4, B. Jain Publishers (P) Ltd. 2008 reprint.

"The Holistic Principles of Ayurvedic Medicine" by Prof. R. H. Singh, ISBN 81-7084-132-6, Chaukhamba Sanskrit Pratishthan 2003 reprint.

Caraka-Samhita, by P.V. Sharma, Chaukhamba Orientalia, Varanasi.

Websites, articles, images:

http://www.wikipedia.org
http://dhanvantari-ayurveda.com
Articles from European Institute of Scientific Research-PDI, The Hague, the Netherlands.

Index

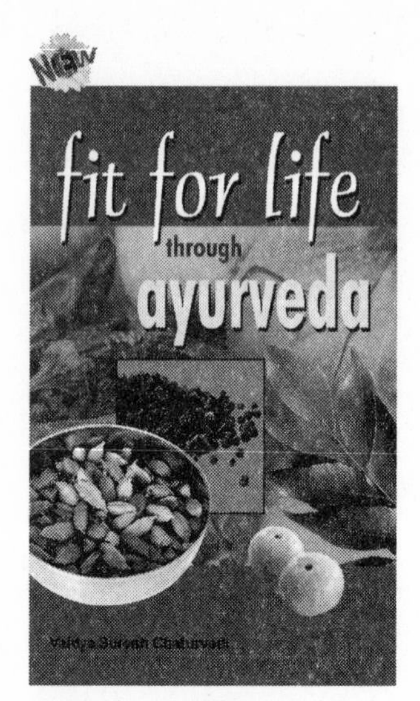

Fit for Life through Ayurveda
Vaidya Suresh Chaturvedi
ISBN 978 81 207 3975 8
₹ 75

Our Series on Secret Guides

Thisjseriesjofjguidesjletsjyoujintoj thejsecretsjofjbetterjhealthjcarej andjalsojgivesjyoujanjinsightjintoj thej causesj ofj diseasesj andj thej waysjtojcurejthemj

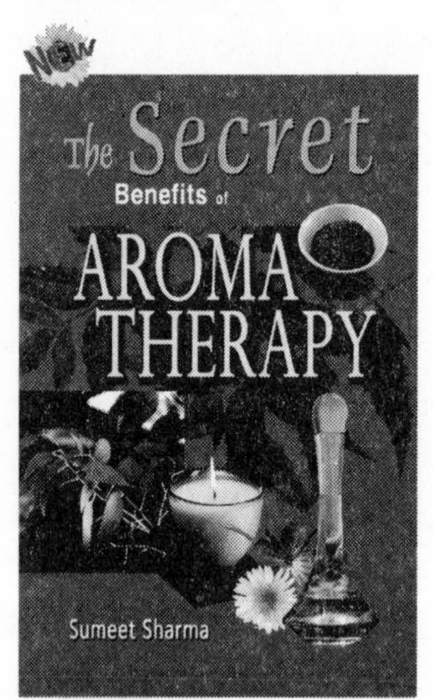

The Secret Benefits of Aroma Therapy
Sumeet Sharma
ISBN 978 81 207 3996 3
₹ 75

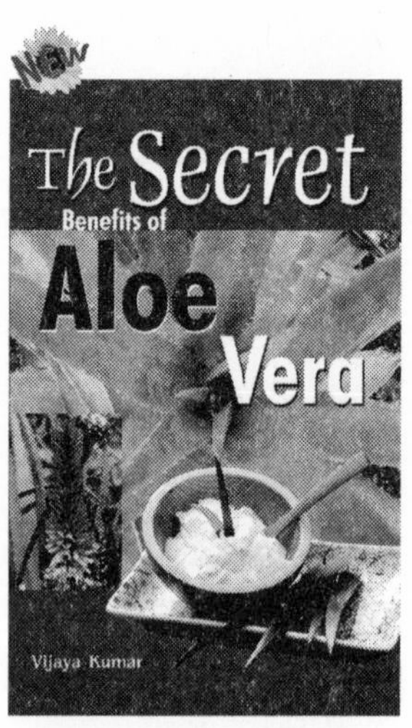

The Secret Benefits of Alloevera
Vijaya Kumar
ISBN 978 81 207 5606 9
₹ 75